CLEAR-HEADED CHOICES IN A SEXUALLY CONFUSED WORLD

By

Terry Hershey

Group Books

Loveland, Colorado

Clear-Headed Choices in a Sexually Confused World

Copyright © 1988 by Terry Hershey

First Printing

For the sake of privacy, all people named in the case studies are composites. Names and details have been sufficiently altered to make them unidentifiable.

Credits
Edited by Nancy M. Shaw
Designed by RoseAnne Buerge

Scripture quotations are from the Holy Bible, New International Version. Copy-right © 1973, 1978, 1984 International Bible Society. Used by permission of Zondervan Bible Publishers.

Library of Congress Cataloging-in-Publication Data
Hershey, Terry.
     Clear-headed choices in a sexually confused world / by Terry Hershey
          p.   cm.
     Bibliography: p.
     ISBN 0-931529-30-1 (pbk.) :
     1. Sexual ethics—United States.   2. Young adults—United States—Sexual be-havior.   I. Title.
     HQ32.H47   1988   88-15700
     306.7—dc19   CIP

Printed in the United States of America

Dedication

To Rich Hurst, friend and fellow journeyer

Acknowledgments

*T*his book is a collection of reflections from my own journey in the area of sexuality and the moral choices all of us make. I owe a great debt to those who, through their friendship or their own writing, have inspired me, challenged me and urged me to clearer thinking in this highly volatile area of life. While I realize that it isn't possible to adequately thank all those who have played a role—not only in the development of my thought, but of my person—I still wish to stop and take a bow to some people who are important to me and who by their life and thought have had an impact on this project.

My thanks to Lewis Smedes, for his personal encouragement and his writing, which helped to create a foundation for my own thinking in the area of choice making. My thanks to Robert Capon and Keith Clark, for the powerful and healing impact their writings had (and continue to have) on my own journey. Thanks to Mike Regele, a friend with whom I walked through the initial stages of thought on the issues of life-giving choices and the distinct decision-making filters, and to whom I am indebted for his contributions in insight and creative thought. Thanks to Tom Thompson, Lewis Rambo, John Westfall, Rich Hurst and Ben Patterson, whose friendships provided for me the necessary foundation of love, support and accountability. And to Norva, my wife and friend, who knows my fault lines, and loves me still.

And to the Group editorial staff, especially Nancy Shaw and Cindy Hansen, for their commitment to seeing the project through to completion.

Contents

Preface

Frog and Toad have a lot to teach us. These two friends are faced with the issue of choices. In a story called "Cookies," we find our friends Frog and Toad faced with an unenviable dilemma—what to do with a large bowl of cookies Toad has made. The best cookies Frog has ever eaten have turned into their present temptation and stumbling block.

> *"We must stop eating!" cries Toad as he eats another.*
>
> *"Yes," says Frog, reaching for a cookie, "we need willpower."*
>
> *"What is willpower?" asks Toad.*
>
> *"Willpower is trying hard* not *to do something that you really want to do," says Frog.*
>
> *How does one find this willpower? Frog and Toad try putting the cookies in a box.*
>
> *"But we can open the box," Toad reminds them. Next they tie string around the box, then they put the box on a high shelf with the help of a ladder. But to no avail.*
>
> *So Frog takes the box outside. He shouts, "Hey birds, here are cookies!" Birds come from everywhere. They pick up all the cookies in their beaks and fly away.*
>
> *"Now we have no more cookies to eat," says Toad sadly. "Not even one."*
>
> *"Yes," says Frog, "but we have lots and lots of willpower."*
>
> *"You may keep it all, Frog," says Toad. "I am going home now to bake a cake."*[1]

I live in a world where sex is an unavoidable and inescapable focal point of our identity. I write about this subject with a mixture of emotions, needs and fears. The generation of which I am a part is more sophisticated, complicated, confused and hurried than the generation of my parents. There is, on the one hand, greater understanding and, on the other hand, more anxiety.

I want to understand this world in which I live, and I want to make healthy choices. My comments about sexuality and the moral choices we make are illumined against the backdrop of my own struggle—a journey of insecurity, experimentation, confusion, failure, guilt, inadequacy, and yes, ecstasy, affirmation and healing. For much of my life I believed I could move on without dealing with or seriously looking at the subject of my body and sexuality. Somehow I separated "me" from my body—all done, of course, with appropriate Christian jargon, believing I had "control of the flesh." I didn't realize how closely tied my person was to my sexuality and to the choices I made.

What was the result? The games I played in my mind had consequences in my body. Because repressed feelings must work themselves out somewhere, those consequences unhealthily locked me into old behavior patterns, dependencies, addictions, fears and denial as I pretended that somehow I was above the struggle.

A part of me still believes that how I handle my sexuality is just my problem. And the reluctance of the church to talk about this and other volatile issues only "fuels the fire." My journey with sexuality—perhaps like yours—has been clouded with confusion, fear, guilt, fantasies, silence, indignance when I feel caught and the belief that no one can really understand. I secretly hoped that all would be resolved when I married, but such was not to be. Like Tom in Pat Conroy's novel *The Prince of Tides,* I "thought I would never think about sex again once I had gotten married or, more precisely, would think about it in connection only with my wife. But marriage had merely been an initiation into a frightening world of fantasy, frightening because of its furious ignition, its secret betrayals, its uncontrollable desire for all the lovely women of the world . . . I longed for constancy, for purity, for absolution."[2]

This dilemma is nothing new. Like me, many young adults find themselves believing one thing and living out another. Some wonder whether their feelings are normal or if some alien force has descended on them. Others find they are using sex for a lot of non-sexual needs—security, attention, power, affection or revenge. When people need all sorts of things from one another, sex can provide one of the most straightforward ways of getting what you need. Many who find themselves lonely and isolated wish for someone to help them understand their struggles while they search for hope and freedom.

I realize that it's dangerous to write about real struggles, real pain and real alienation. Some will view such honesty as an invitation to dwell on negative things; others will shake their heads in disbelief and wonder what's all the fuss about. Some will argue that their sexuality has never been a confusing issue for them. Still others will, like the Levite in the parable of the good Samaritan, turn away from the wounded beside the road to discuss more Christian things, hoping to avoid the worldly subject of sex. These individuals believe that honest dialogue is tantamount to permission for promiscuity. But given that danger, we move ahead. Life today is not for the faint at heart. Now is *not* the time to ignore what is happening in our own lives and the lives of others. Healing can come only with honesty. None of us is an island; and whether we like it or not, we're in this struggle and journey together.

To look honestly at the subject of sex is not an easy task. It means we must be honest with our own journey. And that scares us, especially when we are aware of our own fault lines just beneath the surface. If we're honest, the subject of sex unnerves us all. Feelings of inadequacy, partial memories and a mixture of dread and delight converge to create a climate of uncertain expectancy. Some of us feel obliged to deal with our sexuality like we would a toothache or a noisy neighbor—something that hasn't yet been welcomed as a part of ourselves. "Am I normal?" we wonder. "Can I trust my feelings?" So we come to books, tapes and sermons with the secret agenda that we will find an answer. Inevitably, some will not like what they read. Some will be offended. Some will look for permission. Others will look for ammunition. And still others will merely search for reassurance that they're on the right road.

A real fear is that we may see ourselves and our powerful hunger for relationships and intimacy. We may find those places where we touch each other's lives and actually reach into the secret places of another person's heart and mind. In light of this vulnerability, we face our capacity both to heal and to self-destruct. "Like nitroglycerin," says Frederick Buechner, "[sex] can be used either to blow up bridges or heal hearts."[3]

When Lewis Smedes wrote his book *Sex for Christians,* he recognized this unenviable tension. "Any book on sexual morality is a risk . . . Our sexual nerves weave through the whole fabric of our lives, carrying conflicting messages back and forth from our genitals to our souls . . . So when we talk candidly about sexual morality, few of us can keep our cool."[4]

Where do we turn for perspective? balance? integrity? wholeness? freedom? hope? integration? Like other promises of our time, the temptation for this book—both for me and for you—is that it will promise more than it will deliver. We want to be released from our predicament. We want magic, control, composure. But there is no magic here. This book is merely an invitation to a journey to explore our world, our cultural pressures and our sexuality in light of an affluent, technological, post-pill culture. This journey explores our continued defenses against vulnerability. It asks us to look honestly at how our world affects our decision-making—our addictive cycles, our attempts at control and freedom and our perpetual struggle with willpower and desire. "We must stop eating!" we cry as we continue to reach for the cookies.

In Section One we will look at our belief system and the identity we take to the decision-making process. For decision-making is personal; and the choices we make are identity issues, not just behavioral issues. In Section Two, we will examine a theology of human sexuality. What do we believe, and why do we believe it? We will also look at how our theology affects our moral choices. Section Three

will look at the filters we use to make our moral choices—
the filters through which we process the messages and illusions of our culture, theology and subconscious identity
issues. It is a look at the why behind the what. And in Section Four, we will look at relationship dynamics. Just as
decision-making is personal, it is also relational. Our choices cannot be divorced from our personal and relational
growth. We cannot isolate a moral choice as if it could be
placed in a laboratory vacuum for scrutinization. Morality
is worked out in the context of relationships, and we will
examine how to use those dynamics in all of our relationships.

The task before us is to make moral choices that lead to
health instead of "dis-ease," to freedom instead of bondage,
to wholeness instead of brokenness—in essence, to choose
life instead of death. To begin that process, let's examine
the attitudes necessary for this journey.

•*Humility.* This is not another game of us-versus-them.
The issue of sexuality and moral choices is difficult for all
of us, regardless of the track record of our willpower or the
jewelry worn on our left hand. Humility means confronting
the pride in us that doesn't want to face our inadequacies
for fear of failure or recognizing a need for change. Humility also means rejecting our continued efforts to cover up
our needs and allow others—including God—to lovingly
be a part of this process. With humility we willingly join
the journey of fellow strugglers.

•*Openness.* We will not benefit by hiding or adjusting
the facts. We must confront the illusion that says there are
no moral standards—no rights or wrongs. At the same time,
we need to clearly reject the efforts of those who would
oversimplify the issue of choices by promising a miracu-
lous delivery via a religious experience. There are no
magic wands here. And nothing will be ultimately gained—
save a little comfort—by pretending we are above the issue.
All of us come to this task realizing we stand in the middle
of the battle. Our task is not to run from or avoid that difficult reality.

•*Compassion.* As we walk through the mine fields of
our culture, we need to look at others with compassion. As

we categorize everything into lists for our own moral protection, we need to avoid sacrificing human dignity in exchange for the comfort of moral rectitude and an illusion of personal innocence. Now is not the time to hide behind pious prayer requests for those "in real need." For as we are quick to point out the speck in another's eye, let us also be willing to examine the plank in our own.

•*Confidence.* We need confidence in the Creator's stand for us. It's important to know that we don't struggle alone with this task. We come with a friend, and that friend is Jesus. Because Jesus was fully human and sexual, we can assume he had the same urges we do. Jesus wasn't neuter. Says the author of Hebrews: "For we do not have a high priest who is unable to sympathize with our weaknesses, but we have one who has been tempted in every way, just as we are—yet was without sin. Let us then approach the throne of grace with confidence, so that we may receive mercy and find grace to help us in our time of need" (Hebrews 4:15-16).

One need not be religious, or even Christian, for the reality of the Creator's friendship to be true. God wants us to be whole. He wants us to carve out our sexual ethics in the presence of a loving and holy God who seeks health, not a removed deity who demands his people to maintain a list of rules and regulations. Too often we come to this subject and hear the "you better abstain or die" talk. In reality, we are searching to find the fullness of the Creator's dream for us. We want to express our humanity and sexuality within their healing context, and we want to do this with dignity, health and integrity.

Sometimes I wish life were easier, but I didn't invent it. The truth is that life is difficult. Once we recognize how difficult life is, once we truly understand and accept it, then we will no longer demand to hide behind our need for closure and magic.

Welcome to the journey.

▶ How to Use This Book

To help you with the journey, this book has incorporated reflection and discussion into a series of questions at the end of each chapter. Use those questions for personal reflection and growth. The questions may also help facilitate support groups and classroom discussions. Chapter 12 provides some helpful hints about using this material in small groups.

In addition, there are case studies that can stimulate further discussion and reflection. The case studies reflect real-life situations and offer opportunities for discussions about decision-making filters and the way we approach moral choices. The case studies can be used for teaching tools, role playing or private contemplation.

►SECTION ONE:

Belief Systems

Introduction

Our culture is preoccupied with sex. We laugh about it. We sell cars, perfume and clothes with it. We buy magazines and newspapers that unfurl the latest public scandal involving it. "Did they or didn't they?" we wonder as we wait for the next edition. We listen to talk show hosts casually extol the virtues of sex and prescribe its entertainment value. We keep secrets about it, find ourselves embarrassed in conversations about it, think about it (a lot), feel guilty about it and read bumper stickers on cars about people who "do it higher, deeper and longer" than the uninitiated among us.

But we have yet to come to terms with our sexuality—to be at home with who we are as sexual beings—with our urges, fantasies, confusion, loneliness and vulnerability. We hesitate to stop and ask the difficult questions that lie behind our cultural trappings and behavioral mores.

Culturally—and individually—we are like junior high students smoking their first pack of cigarettes. The moves and language seem self-assured and sophisticated, but something is "out of sync." Although we talk knowledgeably and freely about sex and its techniques, we find that our emotions and relationships are suffering from malnutrition.

► *Our Generation*

We are a part of a generation of adults that's afraid to grow up and, consequently, afraid to make choices. We're a generation caught between two different eras and, therefore, between two different sets of assumptions. Some of our parents were part of the postwar generation that found itself part of an emerging America with its postwar power and affluence, national optimism, patriotism, American work ethic, well-defined social structure and predictable roles for both men and women. All of this optimism balanced itself against the lingering memories of the depression with its lessons about hard work, frugality and caution. Our parents made a conscious choice that life for their children would be rich and rewarding.

Both culture and our parents have encouraged us to express and fulfill ourselves, believing that sheer abundance would somehow support us. We have become the generation with "more"—more education, travel experience, spendable income and advantages than any other generation on Earth. Our parents' dream for the good life for their children was further buttressed by the emerging influence of television and the insidious promise that life comes to those who consume. We grew up believing that our rights included "instant status, important, meaningful work and an unspoiled environment," all displayed among limitless choices such as schools, degree programs, automobiles, home entertainment equipment, TV stations, restaurants, clothing styles, magazines, music styles, churches, vacation opportunities, books and marriage partners.[1] The list seems endless and is complicated even further when we realize that to delay gratification is considered unthinkable. We have been taught to believe that immediate happiness is our right.

With such abundance, why is there still lingering confusion, lack of purpose, relational uncertainty, continued parental dependence and indecision? Gail Sheehy says the motto of this generation is, "Don't lock me in!"[2] As we postpone certain decisions such as marriage, children and careers, they become no's by abstention, creating a pattern in which we make few commitments of any kind. While waiting for the perfect thing to commit to, we have by default become victims in the game of life. As we wait for life to happen, unable to live with any delay in gratification, we dabble here and there. We hope that someone or something will rescue us and provide the meaning we so richly deserve.

► *Choices*

Too many choices? A sense of entitlement? Clouded guidelines? Why, in our affluent, educated, technologically advanced culture, are we so personally, sexually and relationally confused? Numerous magazines and newspapers report that:

- One marriage in two ends in divorce.
- At least 50 percent of all children born today will spend part of their lives growing up in single-parent homes.
- One-and-a-half million fetuses are aborted annually.
- Increasing numbers of couples have decided never to have children.
- Alcoholism affects 25 to 50 percent of American families.
- Family violence touches the life of one woman in every four.

Where did it all go wrong? Susan Littwin says: "It's hard to say when all the experimenting started to turn sinister. It was liberating to drop the Lastex armor of Victorian prudishness and rigid sex roles. It all seemed so harmless, and besides, it's easy to flirt with danger when you have everything. So we started to believe that we had a right to be happy, to be *ourselves* instead of cogs in the wheels of family, community, and friends' expectations."[3]

With our increasing growth in technology and expertise, we have grown more detached about the fundamental changes in our values. We spend our energy concentrating on the skills necessary for continuing this evolution. As one young man remarked, "It's enough just to survive and cover my tail without having to stop and think about why I act the way I do."

Add the church to this search for identity. Baffled at

how to deal with both the issues of young adults and sexuality, it resorts to silence on the one hand and heavy-handed judgmentalism on the other. The church feels intimidated by the fact that it must struggle to find its role. Ironically, many efforts at church programming seem to add only more conflict and confusion. The identity search becomes even more baffling when the church falls in line with the other commodity dispensers who vie for young adults' attention by saying, "Add this activity to your life, and you will be okay."

▶ Our Sexual Identities

How can we possibly sort through these issues that surround the conflict between expectation and reality? Can we come to terms with our identities as sexual beings and our fear of intimacy? Is it possible to understand the moral choices we make in our stress-filled, hurry-up world? This is not a book about *all* choices, only moral ones. Most of the daily choices we face have no moral edge to them at all—what we wear, where we drive or what we eat. Nor is this a book about sexual orientation, sexual technology or sexual dysfunction. It's a book about our identities—the way they've been shaped by the culture in which we live and the way that affects our relationships, our capacity for intimacy and the moral choices we make.

Together we will carefully examine the cultural pressures, unquestioned illusions and personal confusion, as well as our temptation to make this issue "nice and neat" or to seek instant solutions. Honesty, then, is a must for all of us—not just for introspection or scapegoating, but for acknowledging where we are and what we are meant to be.

In this first section, we will focus on understanding our identity and how it has been shaped by the world in which we live. The underlying assumption for this section is that morality is not a behavioral issue, but an identity issue. Unless we recognize and understand that, our morality and identity issues will be decided by default. As we begin to understand our culture's illusions and myths, we begin to recognize and struggle with the addictive cycles we use to substitute sex for intimacy.

CHAPTER 1

Sex and the Choices We Make

*W*e are a wounded generation. Nowhere is this more apparent than in the areas of sexuality and relationships.

We're a generation that has tried to look good, and we've had the tools—money, intelligence, sophistication, advanced technology. But the appearance hasn't worked. For just beneath the surface are the exposed nerve endings of relational and sexual anxiety.

In the words of Woody Allen, "I'm sophisticated. I'm intellectual. I've got angst." Some of us have experienced these same gloomy feelings of anxiety and depression. Our generation is shaped by an affluent, educated, commodity-dispensing culture, living with the aftermath of the sexual revolution and facing the impending possibility of holocaust, via the nuclear warheads from a hostile land or the "silent warhead" (AIDS) within our own culture. Listen to some of the other struggles that exist within our culture today.

■ ■ ■

The tears communicated silent messages of the hurt within. Linda had touched a raw nerve, and she felt her predicament unsolvable. Over the past few months she had tried to forget about it.

Now married four years, this younger-looking 26-year-old wondered aloud whether she and her husband "would ever make it another year." Slowly, she began to talk. "Sex has always been a problem for me. I don't know why; it just has. I mean, I can do it, you know, perform and all that. But it hurts inside. When we're in the middle of intercourse, I start to cry, just shake and cry. I don't know what's wrong with me. I've never had an orgasm. My husband is real tender and patient. He tries to love me in ways he thinks would be enjoyable to me. But . . ." Then she stopped, just to stare.

When asked about her childhood and any experiences of sexual abuse, she paused. "I've never been raped," she responded, "at least I don't think so. But as a child I had many nightmares. My parents were divorced when I was young, and I remember my mom bringing a lot of different men home. My room was next to hers, so I could hear them all night. I remember wanting to scream, 'I hate these men, and I hate my mother for bringing them here!' "

Linda stopped talking, and the tears silently fell.

■　■　■

"What's wrong with me?"

Sandy was 28, single and wondering about her emotional needs. She confided that she had secretly hoped to resolve these concerns by her 30th birthday.

"My friend told me that she thought I give myself away too cheaply." She began to explain,

*and then quickly added lest there be a misunder-
standing, "But it's not like I'm loose or
promiscuous. It's just that I really don't believe
I'm okay. I seem to need someone else to confirm
my value. It's not like I want sex, but why do I
need someone else's arms around me to let me
know I'm loved?"*

■ ■ ■

*They were in love. She was 18; he was an
"older and wiser" 22. Alan and Tina had dated
for four months, and she was pregnant.*

*"What are you going to do?" he asked in a
hurried and frightened voice.*

*"What am I going to do?" she angrily replied,
facing the fear and stark realization that she was
all alone. "I thought you loved me. I thought it
was us. I thought we were planning to get married as soon as you got settled in your new job."*

*"Wait just one minute," he jumped back. "We
never planned on a baby, and you said you were
on the pill."*

*"Oh, so now it's my fault," she fought back,
trying hard to stay defiant in order to avoid
crumbling into tears.*

"Can't you just get an abortion?"

This time there was no response, only tears.

■ ■ ■

*Jeff was a successful 34-year-old man. Be-
sides his strong business record, he had been
married to Lisa for 12 years, had three perfect
children and owned a house in the suburbs. He
was also an elder at his local church and pro-
fessed a strong religious faith.*

*But Jeff was addicted to pornography. At
least twice a week he found himself in a porno
store, looking at the magazines or movies. The*

24-hour period that followed each lapse in will-power was laden with guilt, self-hatred, and promises to himself that he would "never fall again." The painful part of this scenario was Jeff's inability to tell anyone his "secret." He honestly believed that he would meet with judgment and felt there was no hope.

So Jeff lived two lives—as best he could.

■ ■ ■

She was blond, tan and a stereotypical Californian. Outwardly optimistic at age 23, Laura acted like the world was hers. Strong-willed and socially outgoing, she talked with certainty about her views on life. Her parents divorced when she was 8, and Laura found herself without a father. "He's called me twice in the last 15 years," she adds matter-of-factly. She had vowed never to be in a relationship that ended up like her parents.

Now Laura is faced with what might have been. Married at age 19, she separated from her husband a year ago and she talks about her situation. "He still wants to be married, but I can't go back into a situation like that again. He doesn't drink or hurt me, so sometimes I feel guilty for leaving. But the truth is I'm just not happy. And you can't have a good marriage unless you're happy."

After a refill of her iced tea, she goes on. "It was a born-again marriage when we started. But it was like I had to drag him to church. Now he goes every week and preaches to me that what I'm doing is not God's will.

"Is there someone who could love me and make me happy?"

■ ■ ■

"What do you mean you won't leave her?"

Ann asked, looking as if she had just been slapped.

"I can't. You know it. I know it," Tom responded as he toyed with his coffee cup and stared out the window. "My kids even know about us now. And my wife has put down an ultimatum. It's her and the kids—or you. I'm sorry . . ."

"Don't you dare start playing Mr. Family Man on me now," Ann jumped in, interrupting him in midsentence. "For 18 months we've been together. I've put up with holidays without you. I've been stood up because of 'family emergencies.' And I've arranged for our clandestine encounters. Why? Because you promised. You said someday it would be us."

Anger, tears, remorse and humiliation—all began to converge. As Tom reached for her hand she pulled away, unsure of whether she was protecting herself or punishing Tom.

"But Ann," Tom pleaded, "we still have tonight."

■ ■ ■

He died alone. On his death certificate was a brief description—31, male, white, self-employed construction engineer. There was no address, not even a drivers license number. The cause of death was listed as AIDS, but there seemed to be some confusion about that.

A writer for a California magazine wanted to clarify the confusion. He called the man's father, who was listed as next of kin, and asked about his son's death. The father said, "The last time I saw my son, he was unconscious in the hospital. The doctor said he died of a diabetic coma. I don't want to talk about it anymore."

The writer called the doctor to see if he could explain this discrepancy. The doctor apologized, but politely refused to discuss the matter.

A second phone call to the father brought another refusal. Then the conversation ended with a familiar response, "I don't want to talk about this. My son's been gone for a long time."

■ ■ ■

"I don't ever remember it being any different," Tim said, looking like he was straining his memory banks for a new variation on an old theme. At age 36 with dark hair, soft features and a pleasant smile, Tim was now at a place in his life where he had decided to be a little more honest about his sexual orientation.

He continued his line of thinking. "I remember going to parochial school and hearing the lectures about the inherent sinfulness of a homosexual orientation. My response was immediate guilt. I was so sure I was abnormal, that God was going to find some way to punish me. I tried to like women—I really did—but there was never even the slightest attraction. Until my mid-20s, being 'gay' had been my big ugly secret. I was unable to tell anyone, and no one knew. I was lonely and afraid there was something terribly wrong with me. I prayed and read the Bible and went to church, but apparently to no avail. Recently, I've met others who have gone through the same struggle. We've formed a support group, and it's given me permission to believe I may be able to enjoy life again."

Into this uncertain world we walk. Into the world of Linda, Sandy, Alan and Tina, Jeff, Laura, Ann and Tom, and Tim. The concern is more than resolving an academic question by applying a clever formula. Morality must always be in context. The questions, along with the struggles, concerns and fears, take place in real life with real faces and real dilemmas. And that sociocultural context is important.

All of us tend to approach the issue of sexuality, moral choices and human relationships as individual entities—autonomous and independent. We act as if we can have relationships and morality in a vacuum. There is a constant tension between our need for self-discovery and self-sufficiency and our tie to tradition and community. "The irony is that here, too, just where we think we are most free, we are most coerced by the dominant beliefs of our own culture. For it is a powerful cultural fiction that we not only can, but must, make up our deepest beliefs in the isolation of our private selves."[1]

▶ *The Context of Sexuality*

To adequately understand our sexuality, we must begin with our context, history, culture and tradition. Through these windows, we can ask how our sociocultural roots affect our understanding of sex and the moral choices we make.

We are a special generation. "But I don't feel special," one 27-year-old commented to me on hearing this assessment of her generation. "I'm just normal. All I want is a nice house, a meaningful job and a significant relationship, preferably before I turn 30. Is that too much to ask?"

"Yeah," chimed in another, "I'd just like to be happy, that's all."

We are the generation with the "right to be happy." We have more choices than ever before to satisfy our cravings. Our media have presented us with a "sense of entitlement." With this bombardment of choices, it is inevitable that we should become the "postponed generation" as described by Susan Littwin in her book by the same name. Waiting for the "perfect" thing to commit to, we often choose not to commit at all.

This reality is even more evident in the area of relationships, especially with the expanded menu of "more or less equal lifestyles. You can marry; you can have children or not; you can divorce and remarry; you can live with someone who is or is not a lover; you can live alone, with or without a lover; you can be gay or straight; you can even remain married and live separately."[2] In such a shopping mall, where does one turn?

Today's young adults are having more trouble with relationships than almost any other area of their lives. They're afraid of commitment, and they're confused by the number of choices they face. Negotiation of self-interest seems to be the only valid contract for relationships. There are no binding obligations or social understandings to justify a relationship. Relationships exist only to meet two people's needs. Once these needs are no longer being met, the relationship dissolves.

This scenario is not at all surprising. We were born and raised with the non-negotiable nature of our self-sufficiency and expressive individualism. Coupled with our affluence and the advent of a media-dominated culture, we have equated success with consumption. We're told little about success except that we're supposed to get some. And we have no way to recognize it even when it comes. Standards are individual and competitive—linked to money and to "what I possess" (or even "whom I possess").

This crash course with disappointment is examined in *Modern Madness*. Psychologist Douglas LaBier points out that many young adults are restless. "To relieve the stress that has accompanied their success, [these individuals] have embraced everything from aerobics to Zen. But many find they still have the feeling that something is missing."[3] The payoff on the road to success isn't what was promised.

► The Journey

Let's retrace the journey of this special generation.

Our junior high instincts were right. During our pre-puberty naiveté, we needed someone to look up to, someone to admire, someone to mimic, someone to worship, someone to be our hero. The list was long and varied— from Dad to the TV idols, from sports heroes to presidents, from missionaries to rock stars. We had our heroes. We're no longer young and naive. A lot has happened since those junior high years, and we've verbalized our embarrassment over being duped when our heroes couldn't perform.

Our government lied. It waged immoral wars. Our rock stars were drug addicts and several such as Jimi Hendrix and Janis Joplin found life not worth living. Our sports heroes grew older, and our churches gave us a script for life that didn't match the real thing. Even TV ministry gurus scandalized us with their Christianized version of the age-old themes of money, sex and power. We became, as one author put it, "experts in disbelief." The '70s attitude of "trust no one but yourself" bred narcissism. It expressed itself in statements such as "Look out for number one" and "You only live once, so grab all the gusto you can get." Madison Avenue even packaged the quintessence of this age in the magazine called Self.

Heroes became a "luxury"—or at best a pastime—for junior high students. In an era that instructed us to trust no one but ourselves, we cultivated a growing self-absorption, even a protectionism—a world in which ideals were sacrificed at the altar of pragmatics and survival.

And the result? We feel alone. In a sociocultural context—where individualism and individual rights reign—the only acceptable morality between two individuals is whatever they agree is right for them. Of course, the price of this attitude is moral impoverishment. For "just as the notion of an absolutely free self [leads] to an absolutely empty conception of the self, complete psychological contractualism leads to the notion of an absolutely empty relationship."[4]

Our current generation finds itself caught in a paradox. Life hasn't yielded the fruit we expected from our individual retreats. Consequently, our values have remained cloudy, and our selves often empty. There's a tension between protection and survival on the one hand, and the need for an ideal, or something to live for, on the other.

In a recent conversation with a professor at a large California state university, I asked about the causes that motivate the students today. He responded that in the '60s and even the '70s, we witnessed the obvious presence of a cause—be it anti-establishment, peace, anti-Vietnam or "get high." But now the cause is pragmatism. "What do I need to do to get the best opportunities for the best job?"

The jarring conflict between expectation and reality has set in. "As far as most of us can see, there is not any issue that young people in the eighties would find worth fighting for. They prefer not to have a nuclear war, but they would not march about it. They prefer good government leaders to bad ones, but since it is hard to tell which is which, they tend not to vote . . . They can quote fluctuations in the wholesale price of cocaine, but they are uncertain how many senators their state sends to Washington."[5]

It's easy to understand why today's young adults might be motivated by self-interest. Their early years were spent in a society that wasn't quite ready for them. Wars, technology, mobility and American influence made life different from what their parents had experienced in the past.

"This new generation was given so many choices and so few guidelines for making them. They felt they were constantly being asked to pay for other people's miscalculations, sent to clean up other people's messes . . . Their music, their movies, their mores all proclaim this distrust and disillusionment. Why shouldn't I look out for myself? That's what everybody else is doing."[6]

► Cocooning: A Search for Moral Values

In a world where expectations run amok, our coping mechanisms feel the strain. Against the backdrop of affluence, consumerism and the need to be successful, we are confronted with a lingering inadequacy—the feeling that we don't measure up and have no real power to change anything in our world, or even in our neighborhoods. We've truly become experts in disbelief.

Because of the jarring conflict between our expectations and reality, we have discovered that even though we worship at the shrine of the individual, our selves cannot withstand this cultural and internal pressure to be successful, fulfilled, respected and happy. In our public world, all goals are measured by performance and competition, yet privately we yearn for an escape. The result is a growing separation of our worlds. Our public world becomes a forum in which we try to prove our identity, while our private world becomes a way to withdraw. Trend analysts have observed that young adults are more than ever involved in cocooning—the "rapidly accelerating trend toward insulating oneself from the harsh realities of the outside world and building the perfect environment to reflect one's personal needs and fantasies."[7]

In a world where our week provides the stage for our performance and "weekends are made for Michelob," community is seen as an option, used only by groups of people who celebrate a similar lifestyle. The result? Continued withdrawal. Our world becomes even more segmented. Work versus play. Public versus private. Even morality becomes private, a matter of personal preference. The dilemma, of course, is that taken to its logical conclusion, such cocooning leaves all of us as independent islands, each one designing his or her own moral environment. So where do we turn for a determination of values? Who determines the "good"? Ultimately, we're developing a culture in which "being good" becomes "feeling good." How I feel is much more important than how I act, and cocooning is a natural consequence of that kind of ethical process.

▶ Broken Promises: Living Beyond the Sexual Revolution

What happened to the "sexual revolution," that cultural move to see sex as deliverance? This revolution that transported us into the '80s seemed to offer a golden age in which sexual consequences were temporarily suspended. Today we are facing the inevitable price to pay. Indulgence is not easily purchased. This is the age of AIDS and crack, accompanied by death as a convincing ally. We've come face to face with a frightening truth: We're no longer invulnerable. Scientists and their warnings remind us that with AIDS, you're no longer sleeping with just that one person; you're sleeping with everyone he or she has slept with in the latest seven years.

Has it mattered? Recent polls show that at least 25 percent of Americans have changed their sexual habits due to the AIDS epidemic. In truth, "biology has been considerably more effective than the Moral Right in dampening hopes for a utopia of free love."[8] Many people realize that celibacy is no longer a taboo lifestyle. Others hope for a "secondary virginity," another opportunity to start over. Still others don't seem to care. They go on living out the reality that it takes a lot more than biology to put the reigns on lust.

But there is another price tag. It seems our affluence in the area of sex has depreciated in its value. Today's young lovers, who know and talk so much about sex, can't seem to admit their innocence in matters of the heart. Ironically, they are slowly moving toward Aldous Huxley's *Brave New World* where "love," not "sex," was the dirty word. Rollo May's insights about our culture were correct. In 1969 he said, "If our society continued to trivialize sex, to glorify sex objects rather than love, and to equate sexual freedom with happiness, then something dreadful was in store: not an apocalyptic doomsday, but sexual apathy."[9]

Perhaps we think we are exempt from such dynamics. Perhaps we consider ourselves members of an elite group. We are those who, for reasons of conviction, fear or lack of opportunity, have never ventured into the world of expressive sex. Furthermore, we have yet to examine commodity sex where there is a payoff. If we argue from a vantage point of moral superiority and detachment, we miss the point. If we believe we are securely weatherproofed from the storm of sexual ethics, we fail to understand. Our culture as a whole—and that means all of us—lives with the effects of this apathy. We have been numbed by the world in which we live, which inevitably affects our ability to love. How we think about love is central to the way we define its meaning in life, especially in relation to the rest of society. We enter most of our relationships anesthetized. Taught not to feel, we emphasize technique and sophistication, elements that ignore emotions and personal needs. We get the uneasy feeling that our sexual revolution was not a success; it didn't end in victory.

This is not a time to find scapegoats, to say "I told you

so," to keep our heads in the sand or to make moralistic speeches. It's a time for re-evaluation, dialogue and reflection. It's a time to face the truth that into all our freedoms we carry baggage from the past, our personal and cultural limits and weaknesses. Thus, our freedoms may increase our choices, but they guarantee nothing. The issues of our identity and our sense of well-being are still up for grabs.

And so the journey continues. More choices are to be made. But we begin by realizing we don't come to this discussion with clean slates. We bring our stories. We bring wounds and a sense of alienation. We bring our culture and our history. And we bring the expectations of a generation that is learning how to deal with relationships and sexuality in a world where there are too many choices.

▶ Discussion Questions

1. Can you relate to any of the feelings in the stories at the beginning of this chapter? If yes, how do you relate? If no, why not?

2. The author describes this generation of young adults as "special" (page 29). What does he mean? Do you agree or disagree with the description? Explain.

3. How is this generation's postponement of choices (page 29) significant in personal relationships?

4. What are some of the differences of this generation's life journey (pages 30-32) when it is compared with others' life journeys of the past? Have you experienced any of these differences in your own life? If so, how have these differences affected your relationships with individuals from another generation?

5. How has the trend toward cocooning (page 32)— insulating oneself from the realities of the outside world and building a perfect environment to meet one's personal needs—affected your life or anyone you know?

6. Talk about the ways this generation is wounded. What evidence of these wounds do you see around you? List these wounds on a sheet of paper. Think about your own wounds and list these on the same sheet. Pray for God's presence and healing as you begin this introspection.

CHAPTER 2

Illusions About Ethics and Sexuality

"Human beings should never be surprised to be puzzled by their sexuality . . . Sexuality remains one of the prime areas in which persons never get it all together."—Eugene Kennedy[1]

"Are we there yet?" This question was asked a thousand times on every trip my family made, whether we drove to Grandma's house or trekked across the country. And each time it was asked, the level of voice intensity rose and my parents' impatience made itself more apparent by the brevity and staccato of the answer. "No, we aren't!"

That answer was always followed by a recommendation—or was it a plea?—to quiet us. "Why don't you look out the window?" Evidently, my parents failed to realize that we *had* been looking out the window and were tired of that game. Whatever there was to see had been seen and incorporated into a game, contest or school project.

"Are we there yet?"

I have a tendency to look at my sexuality in the same way. "Are we there yet?" In the back of my mind I've as-

sumed there is some place to arrive—a place where all
questions are resolved, discomfort evaporates, confusion is
eliminated and choices are easy. Maybe you think the same
way. We want to say that we've arrived. In fact, one of the
fears of buying or reading this book—let alone being a part
of a discussion group on the subject—is facing the inevitable concerns of those who will wonder whether this area of
sexuality is a problem for us.

Then I wonder, am I—are we—so focused on the destination of this thing called sexuality that we have forgotten
the journey? Are we so tempted to have the right answers
that we forget how to ask the right questions? Are we so
goal oriented, performance oriented or achievement oriented that we miss the process? Are we so concerned that our
sexuality be understood that we have dissected and ana-
lyzed it to the point of detachment?

Most of us have come face to face with what it means to
be sexual beings. The power, unpredictability, allure,
shame, joy, obsessiveness, addiction, sport, conquest, guilt
and pleasure—all weave their way through our minds and
emotions. We are both stimulated and afraid. Of what are
we afraid? We are afraid of our shadow side—our brokenness, incompleteness and vulnerability. Nowhere is our fear
more apparent than when we talk about our sexuality. Neither our trivialization, which reduces sexual behavior to
techniques contained in a 150-page manual, nor our sophistication, which can rise above the emotion of our
sexuality to deliver a level of calm in a cocktail party exchange, has eliminated our fear of being exposed. We want
to be loved. We want to experience the fullness of what it
means to be male or female. At the same time, we fear vulnerability, nakedness and incompleteness.

"Are we there yet?" Where do we begin to unravel the
dilemma of our human sexuality—the approach-avoidance
dilemma within our own bodies? Our tendency is to look
for more precise definitions, as if sexuality is something we
can possess. Our temptation is to go immediately to the didactic portions of the Bible. Perhaps through these moral
injunctions our fears will be calmed by some magical verses, and we will achieve a level of control that reduces the

issue of sexuality to a handout. Many of us go on to teach sexuality as if it is our job to give answers. Unfortunately, I don't have any answers. Sexuality cannot be made "nice and neat," as if it is something that can be controlled, admired and added to our relational résumés. "Nice and neat" just doesn't do justice to real people with real hopes and pain, people with real feelings and passions. People want others who are courageous enough to give them permission to be fully alive even in their incompleteness.

George Leonard, a 63-year-old black belt in aikido, offers these observations about our predicament: "We are in an impatient society . . . For ten years I've had the striking experience of watching students show up the first day with excited eyes, only to drop out quickly at an alarming rate. Only 1 or 2 percent might make it to black belt. Most of the casualties are young men who are mainly concerned with looking good . . . without the necessary long-term practice . . . We've got to accept the fact that mastery . . . is a journey, not a destination."[2]

That's good advice. We need to understand that sexuality is a journey, not a destination. We are tempted to look for a shortcut, a way to short-circuit the process. We want understanding without struggle, relationships without significant emotional investment, joy without pain, love without risk, sex without any strings attached and bodies without the accompanying power of sexual dynamics.

How can we begin to see our sexuality as a journey? Where do we start? What does the journey look like? How do we come to terms with our sexuality as "home" instead of an "alien land"? And when we do come face to face with our sexuality, how can we make choices that are honest, healthy, nurturing and wise? How do we engage in this journey that looks candidly at our sexuality and the choices we consciously or subconsciously make?

I wish this were a simple task, but the world in which we live has already determined the agenda. We cannot begin to investigate this subject with the naive assumption that sexuality can be neatly defined, or that a healthy perspective of ethics naturally follows a comprehension of sexuality. Our primary task is not one of learning, but unlearning. Our task necessarily involves realism. Sexuality and ethics must be rescued from the illusions that have preceded them. This means that our first step in personal growth is honesty about our need for comfort ("Are we there yet?") and about our temptation to find solace in cultural counterfeits such as the illusory promises, or myths, that follow.

▶ *Myths That Cloud Our Perspective*

What are those myths that cloud our perspective? What are the counterfeits that seem so tempting? What are the illusions that prevent us from gaining a healthy understanding of ourselves? I'd like to suggest several erroneous ideas that influence the way we deal with our understanding of ethics and the way we make choices in regard to our sexuality.

1. Ethics, particularly sexual ethics, is understandable in a lecture context or book. It would seem that we believe the purpose of a lecture or a book is to implement the right behavior in the appropriate situation. At a recent young adult conference a pastor asked if he could speak with me just moments before I was scheduled to deliver a series of lectures on the subject of ethics and sexuality. His concern was sincere when he voiced just one question. "You are going to tell them sex is wrong, aren't you?"

The illusion of his question indicated that my lectures would have the power to change behavior. Indeed, I would be the first person to argue about the power of the written or spoken word—to influence, encourage, coerce, manipulate, convince, persuade and impel others to action. And given that reality, an author or public speaker continually faces the uncomfortable realization that his or her words and delivery are a difficult task, not to be taken lightly.

But to say that ethics is a dispensable product capable of being delivered via a carefully crafted sermon, book or workshop is to sacrifice human dignity for the illusion of composure and control. It assumes we can control others' moral choices by language alone. As matters of human sexuality are investigated and diagnosed in half-page articles of People Weekly and half-hour question-and-answer segments with talk show hosts, we realize our approach to human dynamics is becoming more reductionistic. We are the culture that is reducing relational predicaments to five-minute interviews for national news and subject matter for the TV talk show circuit.

Sexual ethics is relationships, which is why I don't recommend reading this book in isolation, putting it back on the shelf and going on with your life. Why? Because community precedes ethics. Our relationships with one another are part of understanding this process. We are human only when we are in relationship to other humans. Consequently, we are ethical only when we are involved in relationships with others. Virtue, nurture, tenderness, care and love have meaning only within a relationship. Ethics is carved out of the journey of community—out of the dialogue, the struggle and the modeling where we create for each other mirrors of encouragement, support, impetus, forgiveness and conviction.

Only within community can we see ourselves clearly. For in community, the ideal system—proposed by the well-crafted and well-meaning book or sermon—sooner or later (usually sooner) gives way to the reality that humans are not perfect. Believing the right things is important, but it's not enough. Belief must be translated into "everydayness," where black and white dissipate to confusing shades of gray, where kisses aren't contracts of commitment, where best intentions almost always fall short, where willpower is elusive and where faith in God doesn't always guarantee easy choices and storybook endings.

Says Eugene Kennedy: "The sooner we can live with the fact that we are never going to be perfect the more surely we will deal with our sexuality in a satisfying and enriching way. If we allow ourselves to be fallible and forgive ourselves and others for this, at least half of our troubles disappear."[3] If moral choices are to be understood in a cognitive context alone, then our temptation will be to seek comfort through understanding ("I think I've finally got a handle on my sexuality") and the accumulation of right answers ("You're going to tell them sex is wrong, aren't you?"). At this point ambiguity becomes the enemy. We begin to seek an accumulation of knowledge and so-phistication, better formulas, more precise techniques and a newer awareness for us to hide behind, but it doesn't work. Why? Because when we're honest with ourselves, we must agree with Andrew Greeley's observation that "no matter how sophisticated or how mature or how self-possessed or how casual or how cool we may think our approach to sex-uality is, we are all of us basically boys and girls at the beach."[4]

2. Our sexuality can be domesticated. Our desire for control and personal security will find a way to attempt to tame our sexuality, to bring it under control. Questions about this myth are typical. "Why did God give me such a big appetite for sex if he meant for me to starve?" "Why is it far more exciting to fantasize about the women I work with than to make love with my wife?" "Why is it that on some days I can handle my sexual drives, but on other days it's as if I'm trapped in someone else's body?" "Why is it so difficult to say no?" "Why is it that even though I say my sexuality is not an issue, when I get close to a per-son of the opposite sex I become anxious and aloof?" All these questions about sexuality can be answered the same as the following question:

"Why does the largest mammal in the world, the sperm whale, have such a small throat?"

The answer? "Because that's the way it is and there's really nothing you can do to change it."

There's something about our Western mind-set that as-sumes we can understand any enigma, dilemma or predica-ment. It is assumed that we can simply reduce any issue to manageable components and apply our expertise. The as-sumption that all of life can be reduced to manageable components for us to analyze, categorize, label and manage is a purely cognitive approach to life. Questions are raised only for the answers that will be given. Life is controllable;

therefore, it is possible and necessary to "get our act together."

This attitude strips life of mystery. When there is no wonder about how life operates, there is only frustration over unresolved quandaries. We are afraid to say, "I don't know." When we refuse to acknowledge mystery, we also refuse to accept creativity. The irony of this position, of course, is that it is the "eros," or sensuous, part of our lives that summons us to creativity. When the act of love invites us to the joys of the creative process, we are often caught up in fear and guilt and refuse the invitation. "We learn not to surrender to the erotic but to use it—as a means of conquest and exploitation, as a way of measuring performance, of reducing tension. Then, when boredom inevitably overtakes us, we look for new lovers or new techniques. We seek advice from experts, sure-fire solutions to our problems."[5]

Sure-fire solutions? Life is lived with the inevitable "if only"—hoping that an answer is only around the corner. But what if our sexuality is an invitation to the ambiguity of life, and not an impetus to seek relief via cognitive control or mastery of technique? Andrew Greeley reminds us: "The most fundamental insight that primitive man had about sexuality is one that we frequently overlook or forget: that it is a raw, primal, basic power over which we have only very limited control . . . Living with sexuality does not mean eliminating its primal force; it means, rather, understanding how primal the force is and channeling it in directions which are both socially and personally productive."[6]

My unresolved sexuality becomes something I am afraid of. Consequently I avoid real feelings, repress actual needs and evade honest personal dialogue. I feel abnormal. "Something's wrong with me!" "Maybe someday I'll be over this 'confusion.' Someday I'll understand." "Maybe I'll be able to control my sexual feelings with better discipline. Maybe someday it will all make sense."

The result? We come to life—and consequently our sexuality—attempting to divide ourselves into manageable components that we can study and control. And as long as ambiguity or mystery is viewed as the enemy, there can never be an invitation to embrace ourselves for who we are—sexual, human, incomplete and needy. There is no permission to revere the gift of life, the essence of the unknown. For as Bernard Ramm, a theologian, once remarked in a lecture, "Spirituality is the ability to live with ambiguity."

3. If we are Christian, then it is easier to maintain our ethics. Or, "If I were really committed, my life would be easier." This illusion is subtle and pervasive. And those of us who teach project our own sense of guilt onto those we teach by nurturing this illusion. This myth is just another variation on the illusion of control—that somehow I have the power to make life easier. Couched in religious language, the issue sounds like a faith question. "If only I had more faith." Do we expect God to give us our faith and an easy life in exchange for a good performance or services rendered?

What's at stake here? What am I afraid of? Why am I so tempted and entrapped by this illusion? Where's the power behind this simple "if only"? I want to look good. I want you to think well of me. I want to have a competent reputation. Why? Because being significant is important. When I am done on this earth, I want it to be said that Terry mattered. My world teaches me that people matter when they have some pragmatic value, some achievement or some goods for barter. My normal and necessary need for significance is clouded with the cultural interpretation that my significance is measured by my performance. It's no wonder my approach to ethics has been adulterated by the cultural philosophy of accumulation.

In religious language it sounds this way: "If I had more faith, I would have more control over my life." Or, "If I had more faith, I wouldn't have to struggle with any decision-making in the area of sexuality." The irony of these statements is that our continual emphasis upon faith performance only reinforces the insidious misconception that our identity is linked to our ability to control or perform. It subtly alienates us from our sexuality and our humanness. We deny doubt, we fear being ordinary and we reject anything that hints of our fragile nature. We feel punished, somehow abandoned by God, for our weakness. We pray, read and listen and then wonder why there's no relief. And, in turn, we project our fear of inadequacy onto those around us, using a more rigid and judgmental approach to issues of sexuality. We hope that our position of judgment will defend us against our true sense of vulnerability and weakness.

4. Morality is built on a hierarchical system; some sins are worse than others. We don't exactly come right out and say it's better to be accused of gluttony than lying. And lying, if it's for a good cause, seems less severe than misappropriation of funds. But being divorced is worse, and being accused of sexual sins receives top billing on the church scandal review.

There's a good example from an old movie. The scene went something like this: A man steals a set of tools from his place of employment for his best friend's birthday. However, when his friend asks him to lie to his wife while he has an affair, he refuses because he says, "It would be wrong."

"Wrong?" the friend responds in anger and surprise. "You, who can steal tools from the factory, have the audacity to lecture to me about wrong?"

"Yeah, well, that was a factory. This is personal."

Another example happened to me. While attending a workshop titled "Ministering With Persons in Extramarital Affairs," the emphasis became clear. This well-researched and fairly insightful information was for us (the listeners) to help those "in need." This dynamic created a false sense of security for those of us who attended the workshop. It seemed that somehow we (the lucky ones) were above any struggle. And it was our job to help those with needs.

We cannot lull ourselves into a false sense of security, with an artificial us-versus-them delineation. The issue of sexuality and moral choices is a challenge to all of us. Our ability to make healthy choices is predicated on our willingness to face our membership in the human race. That includes recognizing our fault lines, those ready reminders of our own fallibility.

"Are we there yet?" The temptation to short-circuit is real. Our journey toward health and wholeness must be built on a foundation of continual honesty about the illusions that derail us.

In a world where young adults have been raised to model the ultimate man or woman—fit, trim, lively, independent, career minded, alone, no spouse, no clinging children—we need permission not to run from our humanness—our incompleteness and our neediness.

In a recent Peanuts cartoon, Charlie Brown sat in front of the psychiatrist booth. Lucy sat in the booth charging a nickel for her services. She began expanding eloquently about life. "Life, Charlie Brown, is like a deck chair."

"Huh?" he responded.

"Some people put their deck chair on the front of the ship so they can see where they are going. Some put their deck chair on the rear of the ship so they can see where they have been. On the cruise ship of life, Charlie Brown, which direction is your deck chair facing?"

Said a meek Charlie Brown, "I haven't figured out how to get mine unfolded yet."

There's a little of Charlie Brown in all of us. Maybe we need permission to believe it. For if we no longer need to maintain the illusion of control, we're free to continue the journey.

▶ **Discussion Questions**

1. When we approach our sexuality as a "journey" rather than a "destination," the way we view our sexuality is changed (pages 38-40). Explain how this statement applies to your own life.

2. Think about ways we hide behind the myth that ethics can be learned through lectures or books (pages 40-42). Talk about the way you see others hiding behind this myth. How do their actions affect them? How do their actions affect others? After listening to others talk about ways people hide behind this myth, can you see yourself in any of these descriptions? Why or why not?

3. How do you attempt to domesticate your sexuality (pages 42-44)? Talk about the one attempt to "control" your sexuality you see most evident in your own life.

4. What happens when we project and accept the image that moral choices are easier to make if we are Christians (pages 44-45)? How does this myth affect our relationships with others? How does this myth affect our relationship with God?

5. Which myth has most affected your way of thinking about morality and sexuality? In what way? What did you learn about this myth in your reading and discussion? You may wish to share your ideas with a friend and ask him or her for support as you struggle with these new thoughts.

CHAPTER 3

Decision-Making: Who Owns Me?

"One way to express the spiritual crisis of our time is to say that most of us have an address but cannot be found there."—Henri Nouwen[1]

We have received an invitation to a journey. That's what morality is all about, and so is the Christian faith. Both experiences are based on a journey and a process. It's not where we have arrived ("Are we there yet?"), but the direction we are going. It's not a possession or an asset for public approval ("Look at how moral he is"), but a relationship with ourselves, God and the world around us.

Morality is personal. We cannot divorce our choices from who we are as individuals. It would be easier to approach ethics like a scientific experiment. Then we could objectively analyze and evaluate it from a safe distance, use the dissected behavioral carcass as a prop for discussion and dispose of those parts we don't want to deal with. Morality could be decided by majority rule. We could decide our ethics by opinion polls and majority elections and display the results on brightly colored graphs in national newspapers.

But morality is not that easy. All of us carry the wounds of misguided promises, unrealistic expectations and squandered opportunities. All of us experience lonely nights, broken dreams, wasted good intentions and subconscious (and sometimes overt) acts of self-destruction. All of us are capable of such extremes. But most of us have learned to control ourselves against such excesses, especially when we consider our need to maintain an appropriate image. And for the most part, we're considered stable and well-behaved, not to mention respectable. But when we are alone—and lonely—we catch glimpses of the "real us," the things that obsess our thoughts, our secret wishes, our capacity to be harmful and injurious and the things that might have been.

To understand morality and my own sexuality, I must come face to face with me. Why is that frightening? Because I'm not sure I'll like what I see. Because if I'm honest, I will realize that I am—in the words of C.S. Lewis—a "bundle of self-centered fears, hopes, greeds, jealousies, and self-conceit, all doomed to death."[2]

Does this sound negative? I don't think so, especially when my alternative is to treat my sexuality as if there were no shadow side. It is to assume that my moral choices can be implemented by correct theology, good intentions and a strong will. It is a position from which I can moralize about others (who are worse off, of course), justify my own behavior ("But there's a reason") and repress any confusion or fear that may surface. I can remain detached and hope that my underlying emotions will never be exposed. But underneath such an exterior, I must constantly be aware of my tendency to disguise the truth about myself.

▶ Sexuality and Behaviorism

A relatively common philosophy says that sex (and sexuality) is strictly a behavioral issue. This idea detaches us from the personal nature of our moral choices—and the shadow side of our motivations. We find this concept stated in its pure form by behaviorist H.J. Campbell: "Sex is not inextricably involved with marriage or any other social institution. It is simply a form of sensory pleasure-seeking."³

While many would take exception to Campbell's definition, they nonetheless live their life by the same underlying premise—namely, that moral choices are strictly behavioral. From B.F. Skinner's behavioral psychology to Christian fundamentalism, the emphasis is the same: Ethics is what you do or don't do. In the case of behaviorists, what you do (or don't do) is for personal pleasure. In the case of fundamentalists, what you do, or more realistically, what you don't do, is for personal purity. These two ideas are similar because there is a common illusion of personal control.

We "assume that the problems of sexuality can be solved in terms of who you sleep with and what particular organs are combined in what ways. As anyone who has pondered his own sexual experience seriously knows, it is not all that easy—and it never will be so long as man has both a fantasy life and the power to interpret and give meaning to his behavior."⁴ In other words, we err if we assume that ethics is strictly behavioral.

At one level I suppose that assumption is okay. The Christian behavioral approach assumes the human personality is one-dimensional, a "what you see is what you get" approach. While denying the subconscious world of thought, fantasy and feeling, this approach views the human condition as static and non-developmental. But in truth, all of us continue to be influenced by the unconscious, a vital part of our personalities. This unpredictable influence adds mystery to our lives that we can never understand if we continue to consider only our behaviors.

It's safe, of course, to treat our personality and humanity as a spectator and bystander. In this way, we avoid the inevitable contradiction of "who we want to be" and "who we really are." Instead, we feel anxious about our attempt to maintain a semblance of composure.

Our behavioral approach also significantly affects the way we counsel others, whether as a cleric, a lay counselor or an interested friend. As a result of our own preoccupation with behavioral control, we tend toward easy labeling, moralizing and a general need to fix our friend's or client's problem. The prevalence of this behavioral approach is evidenced by the glut of magazine articles and books that line bookstores' shelves, promising answers with yet another catchy how-to title. *How to Make Love to a Man, How to Overcome Depression, How to Meet Girls Without Really Trying*, and the list goes on. There is nothing wrong with thinking clearly about the issue of sexuality and the moral choices we make. Our impatience to resolve the issue, however, by attaching labels of moral judgment, prescribing a laundry list of cure-all recommendations or enjoining individuals toward more prayer does little to deal with the real and underlying anxieties individuals face.

In our eagerness to be a friend or a counselor, we may judge or deal with the act rather than listen for the person's life struggle. If we can withhold moral judgment, we will hear much more, including why a person is using his or her sexuality as a way to take care of the inner pain that needs to be healed.

There is more to understanding sexuality and the choices we make than simply confronting the present sexual conflict. We do not solve the problem by getting someone to stop, by helping him or her think of something else, by offering appropriate discipline or confrontation or by providing clarity and understanding. We are dealing with more than delinquent behaviors, lingering adolescent fantasies or perversion; we are dealing with people—whole people. And our approach to both sexuality and ethics must be one that addresses the whole personality with its range of complex and confusing needs, motivations, fears and dreams. It's easy to recognize the compartmental approach to sexuality when people respond to my offer to read a book or attend a seminar on the subject of sexuality by saying, "Sounds great, but it's not an area in which I'm having problems."

It's not the purpose of this book to solve problems. It's our purpose to continue the journey of self-understanding and self-acceptance. To do that, sexuality cannot be compartmentalized. I am reminded of an incident that happened at a workshop I was conducting in southern California. About halfway through the day, one woman near the back raised her hand and began to voice an objection. "I am really frustrated with this workshop. You seem to be talking only to the people in the room who 'do it.' What about those of us who don't 'do it'?"

I realized immediately that she had compartmentalized sex. She assumed sexuality and the choices we make about our sexuality are linked only to what happens with our genitals. My response to her was: "I'm afraid I have miscommunicated. At any time during the last four hours did you touch another person? Did you smell anyone's perfume? Did you feel anger or frustration or relief? Did you laugh or cry? Did you hug anyone or wish to be hugged? All of those emotions and sensations are part of what it means to be human and therefore sexual. Understanding sexuality and its choices permits us to learn to be at home with ourselves and with another person. As a result of this understanding, we can learn to make healthy choices."

Another problem with the behavioral approach is that doing the right things for the wrong reasons doesn't make you pure or righteous or healthy. During the time of the New Testament, there was a group of "behaviorists" known as Pharisees. The Pharisees discovered that Jesus believed there was another level to morality. In fact, Jesus bluntly warned his followers, "Unless your righteousness surpasses that of the Pharisees and the teachers of the law, you will certainly not enter the kingdom of heaven" (Matthew 5:20). On a behavioral model, that statement seemed impossible because the Pharisees were known for their behavior. They had set the standards for uprightness and rectitude; well-behaved, obedient and stable commonly described these religious leaders. Jesus' point, however, was relatively simple—your morality must go deeper than your behavior. It must somehow touch your heart, identity and belief system.

▶ The Heart of Morality: Our Identity

Morality is not based on what you do; morality is based on who you are. The issue is not being good or bad, but being free—learning to be at home with yourself. An advertisement sponsored by the Humane Society graphically illustrated this principle. The ad featured a full-page, color picture of a puppy and kitten and encouraged people to open their homes to these homeless animals. As an emotional pull, it worked. But it was the sentence over the top of the puppy and kitten that caught my eye. It simply declared, "It's who owns them that makes them important!"

In the same way, our moral choices are built on the base of "who (or what) owns us." In this case, identity and intimacy—not sexuality—are the primary issues. My decision-making with regard to my body and genitals becomes clouded when I fail to understand my needs, my addictions and my relentless drive for intimacy. Without stopping to take an inventory of the self, I become easy prey to the unspoken promises of the culture in which I live and to the comfortable illusion of seeing life as behavior only.

The question now becomes, "Who or what owns me?" Therein lies the impetus behind our decision-making. To answer that question requires honesty and healthy introspection. I can be owned by my need to be needed, my need to rescue, my addiction to the high of a sexual experience, or even my addiction to the high of conquest. I can also be owned by my need to be held, my need to prove my masculinity or femininity, my need to "screw up" to prove my unworthiness, my need to be a doormat in someone else's life or my need to be powerful. In coming to terms with this area of neediness, we begin to successfully address the issue of our decision-making. For change cannot and will not be effective if it is strictly behavioral; it must touch who I am, which includes my fears, drives and needs.

▶ Morality and the Addiction Cycle

I come to this place in the book with my own history as the impetus to uncover an understanding of decision-making that goes beyond the behavioral model. I am an adult child of an alcoholic. And the reality of that fact impacts who I am today and how I make my decisions—or who owns me. While I am aware that not everyone can relate to being the adult child of an alcoholic, there are some principles of human behavior and decision-making that affect us all. For the culture that creates excessive addiction cannot scapegoat the alcoholic or the drug addict for all the relational ills of the day. The problem runs deep and affects us all; it is the reality of an addictive culture.

Recently, much has been written about addiction and its epidemic proportions in this country. (See the Bibliography in the back of this book.) We need to take advantage of this research and the insights it has provided, for it gives us some cognizance of the cultural dynamics that impact the decision-making of young adults in today's world. Evidence verifies the fact that our lives have been shaped by an addictive culture. How that culture impacts us, the world in which we live, the choices we make, the relationships we build and the way we listen, counsel and teach is for us to explore further in this book.

What do we mean when we talk about addiction, an addictive culture or an addictive system? In his book *The Freedom We Crave*, William Lenters provides a helpful backdrop to our discussion. Addiction is, he says, the "drama of the human spirit responding to the stress of life."[5]

We are a culture responsive to immediate gratification, easily enslaved by the "pleasure carrot" that promises enhancement, ecstasy or fulfillment. And we are made all the more susceptible in a culture that isolates the individual as self-sufficient. As we are indoctrinated with the "Madison Avenue" dogmas that reinforce immediate gratification, ecstasy and the right to happiness, the cycle continues.

Our culture inculcates all of us in a disease called the addictive process—described by Anne Wilson Schaef as a process "whose assumptions, beliefs, behaviors, and lack of spirituality lead to a process of nonliving that is progressively death-oriented."[6]

To understand sexuality and the moral choices we make, we must contend that none of us is exempt from this addictive process. Lenters says: "All have fallen short of the freedom we crave . . . The addiction experience is the human experience, not the monopoly of a boisterous or boozy 10 percent of the drinking population. We all weave our own behavior patterns and habitually repeat that which provides and secures relief and escape . . . Because everyone seeks safety, salvation, purpose, and meaning, we are all vulnerable to the addictive process."[7] Like Frog and Toad, our friends from the Preface, we seem caught between wanting something that is good and not knowing when or how to say no. Like the mosquito attracted to the "bug light," which will eventually kill it, we too find ourselves attracted to behaviors, obsessions and preoccupations which will, if unabated, lead us to death.

For clarification, we must note that not everyone is an "addict"—an individual who is diagnosed as dependent upon an outside stimulus. Unfortunately "addict" can become a catchword or cliché. But all of us without exception are affected by a system—a way of life, a way of thinking, a culture—that is addictive. To understand the full picture of moral choices in the '80s and '90s, this is a dynamic we must not overlook.*

Addiction means we buy into a life cycle that takes care of our wounded and inadequate identity. It's necessary because we're afraid to risk the possibility that we may be okay, even though we are human and incomplete. Our survival mechanisms only perpetuate a false self.

Why are we susceptible to this addictive process? Because our false self is built on a thinking disorder, a faulty belief system that fears non-acceptance or even abandonment if our humanness is revealed. Inevitably, when we repress our real feelings, our subconscious becomes a powerful force that must be reckoned with on our journey to self-discovery. For what is repressed will eventually own us if we do not deal with it directly.

---

*It's not within the context of this book to explore specific questions and issues that determine individual addiction; however, it is important to the thesis of this book that all of us are impacted by the addictive (compulsive) nature of our culture. That's important because it allows us to explore the identity currents underneath our moral decision-making. Indeed, there are an increasing number of people who are "clinically addicted"—that is to say, their identity is dependent upon an object, a person, a chemical or some form of acting out sexually, and they are literally no longer in control. I strongly recommend further reading in the following books: *Out of the Shadows* by Patrick Carnes; *Women Who Love Too Much* by Robin Norwood; *The Freedom We Crave* by William Lenters; *A Time to Heal* by Timmen Cermak; and *Co-Dependence* by Anne Wilson Schaef.

Then what is it we are hoping to take care of by involving ourselves in an addictive cycle? No matter what addiction we choose—alcohol, drugs, stealing, busyness, eating or even church—there is an attempt to find relief from pain or negative feelings. Relief becomes even more difficult when we make the morality issue strictly a behavioral one. Examine the following chart and its observations on how addictive cycles operate. Think about your own addictions, those things you continue to use to relieve your own pain or negative feelings.

Chart of an Addictive Cycle

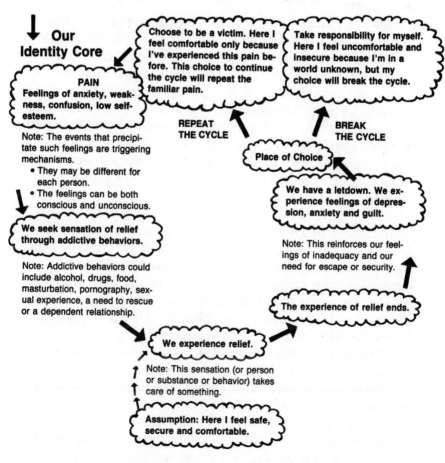

Addiction is the human condition, and it's not new. In the New Testament, Paul shared his own struggle when he lamented: "I do not understand what I do. For what I want to do I do not do, but what I hate I do" (Romans 7:15). This is the reality of sin. We are creatures whose paradise is lost. At creation, humans were given the power that comes from freedom—the freedom we have to enjoy, the freedom to say no, the freedom to trust. What we didn't understand was that this freedom was based on our identity being intact. We didn't need to prove anything to anyone with our choices or even with our right behaviors. We were free to live within the reality that there was nothing to prove, earn or pursue. We were free precisely because we were owned by someone.

All freedom is contingent freedom as opposed to absolute freedom. In other words, I'm free to make this choice because I'm no longer free to make another choice. That which owns me defines my freedom. We've all seen the "bowl of cookies," and for us, contingent freedom isn't enough. We want "absolute freedom." Lenters says: "We willfully step out into the empty space created by the fantasy of absolute freedom. It's a stunning view, but there is no breathing room. In a panic to survive . . . we grab on to anything that promises us breath, even if for only a few moments."[8]

Our culture only intensifies the addictive cycle. As young adults in a society that places a premium upon immediate gratification, they are confronted with how to extricate themselves from this tangled web. The addictive cycle encourages emulating "lifestyles of the rich and famous." The cycle is energized by consumerism and sees the weekend escape as a model for all of life and relations; it's no wonder we are a culture consumed by addictions. Alcohol, drugs, romance, success, religion and the American dream are all variations on the same theme.

What does all this mean to our discussion? Let's take a look at two practical implications.

One, it means that "there are no cure-alls, no offers of grace without responsibility, no easy 'how to's,' no moralisms to help you on your way. You will not discover the secret of how to be your own best friend or to pull your own strings."[9] We can be so focused on the symptoms that we miss the cause, and the result is inappropriate advice, moralistic detachment or an inordinate optimism regarding our own willpower.

For our discussion in this book to be healing, we must first take a realistic look at our predicament of powerlessness. Our obsessions and addictions—those things that own us—have rendered us powerless and choiceless. Our culture is at the mercy of that which titillates (How else can we explain society's incredible preoccupation with the details of events such as the affairs of political leaders or the demise of religious empires?), of that which offends (Why else would some preachers denounce pornography with accusations that are more erotic and arousing than the pornography itself?), or of that which gratifies (Is the only way to sell a car with a sexy, half-clothed man or woman on the hood or behind the wheel?).

Two, our healing as individuals and as a nation can come only with honesty. The biblical concept of honesty is "confession," which literally means "to take responsibility for." When we take responsibility for who we are now, for the choices we have made and for the consequences of our choices, we will reap the benefits of a healthy inventory and a hard introspection. We will look directly at who owns us.

► *To Whom Do I Belong?*

Let's begin that healing process by looking at several cultural promises, personal fears and a combination of distortions that own us. Those addictive survival mechanisms perpetuate a false self and affect the way we approach life, the moral choices we make and the way we shape our view of God.

1. The performance principle. Our identity is inextricably tied to how we perform—to what we do and to what we do better than most. It's a cultural message that is both enslaving and intoxicating. It's a part of the addictive process.

We are no longer a culture of lovers; we are technicians. Preoccupied with the size and shape of our bodies, multiple orgasms and meaningful foreplay, we emerge from our sexual encounters—whether real or fantasies—straining to see the judges' score cards held high like those at a diving meet. Our identity is linked to how well we have performed. In a culture where impotence is so feared, it's no wonder the number of people who have experienced, or do experience, either impotence or frigidity continues to rise.

We hear the message, "Orgasm is life." "Having one" is the issue. It doesn't matter how, just whether. But orgasms really have little to do with love. Those who insist on evaluating every sexual performance have already failed the test.

The irony is that our culture has prided itself in seeing the evolution of the "sensitive male." But we have only added this accomplishment to our list of relational performances, as if we are encouraging one another to "do sensitivity." When our emotions seem to call for stagelike performances, we become detached and lose our sense of connectedness. We begin to fear that we may have to deliver in love those things we promised in lovemaking. Our sensitivity is threatened by our inability to be real and vulnerable and incomplete.

In a culture that advertises an enlightened view of human relationships—feeling, responsiveness and tenderness—why are we still so preoccupied with performance? Why do our movies grow more violent and our pornography more perverse? We live in a culture where it's necessary to look good. Image becomes important. We try to make others see us as we want to be seen and honestly believe we can control others' impressions. Consequently, our real feelings are repressed for fear they will not measure up or be acceptable. Psychiatrist Lyon Hyams has observed the powerful dynamic of this cultural illusion with adolescents. He describes it as the need for "external and absolute criteria to measure feelings and performance."[10] It is a tyranny of perfectionism, requiring a sophistication that fears being

ordinary. When relationships become incapable of true communication and become disposable, we realize they are
built on a foundation of win or lose.

2. A cure for loneliness. We are all afraid of isolation.
And while we may often wish to be a rock or an island,
the wish is self-protective. There are those times when we
wish we never had to cry or feel any pain. It's a part of
our relational dynamics. We want relationships—talking,
touching, caring, listening, needing—but we are at the
same time afraid. And we approach our relationships with
the same caution and sterile objectivity with which we
approach matters of science. Guilty until proven innocent, we find that we rarely commit ourselves fully, and
we wonder why relationships inevitably fail or come
up short.

Sex, in a range of physical or genital expressions, becomes a way to short-circuit the process. Self-protective
and afraid to care and commit, we dance around the issue
by making excursions with our bodies. We somehow assume the body is free from the approach-avoidance enigma
that our mind and emotions go through. "What if I commit
myself to him and then find I've made the wrong choice?"
"I always feel my own identity gets swallowed up by the
woman I'm with. I'm going to wait to commit." In another
form of compartmentalization and detachment, we engage
in lifestyles that only exaggerate our predicament. We secretly hope our bodies will not suffer the consequences of
fear and pain that would result from an emotional
commitment.

And so it is that our bodies become our only language
of intimacy. Or, in the words of one young woman, "When
lovers run out of things to say, they speak with their bodies." The addictive nature of this illusion is clear, but it's
not easy to admit or overcome. For we are victims of the
promise that there is a solution to our loneliness without a
severe cost to our self—or emotions. In the end we discover we have been conned into believing that our bodies are
detached from our emotions. We've also been conned into
believing there's an easy solution or an answer to our

loneliness.

Too many people put their sexual relationships before friendships. But sex is only temporary. When it's over, people still need individuals with whom they can talk. Sexual interludes offer moments of closeness but no long-term solutions to the problem of loneliness.

The myth is that loneliness is a solvable problem. Because we are a culture of expertise and answers, no problem escapes our capacity to solve it. Inevitably, we run from incompleteness. And loneliness, which is a sign of our incompleteness, must be avoided, assuaged, eluded or disdained. Some of us even become addicted to our method of escaping the human condition through outlets such as sex, eating or watching television.

3. The display of power. Here we find a close relationship between sexuality and hostility. This combination is almost always destructive. At the root of this unmet need is a low sense of self-esteem, resulting in relationships that attempt to reinforce some sense of okayness.

This inner wound may result from several reasons—a preoccupation with a need to prove one's worth, an undernourished childhood and an incessant need and inability to get attention, or an accumulation of unresolved anger and hostility (against parents, friends, members of the opposite sex or life itself) that requires some revenge or personal vindication. Whatever the reason, the result is manipulation.

It's important to note that many people—mostly males—enter marriage relationships with a Christian behavioral view of sex and therefore perceive that any sexual activity within that marital bond is right or okay. The consequence is that a lot of sex exists to meet non-sexual needs—namely power—that is not at all healthy or healing to the relationship. But because of their "correct theology," no change is deemed necessary even at the expense of human dignity.

Even though this wound is often subconscious, it is nevertheless real. Sex becomes both a weapon and a shield, a way of staying in control. Sex also becomes a way to be strong, invincible and powerful. It offers a way to get even with life, a way to prove, a way to chalk up another notch in the belt, a way to disrupt the cycle of giving and receiving—especially if one is afraid of receiving. We use sex so we can maintain our position of power.

4. The lure of romance. The addictive distortion of the power of romance is evidenced in the success of recent books such as *Do I Have to Give Up Me to Be Loved by You?* and *How to Break Your Addiction to a Person.* In the second book, author Howard M. Halpern notes that "people, in droves, choose to remain in their prisons, making no effort to change them—except, perhaps, to hang pretty curtains over the bars and paint the walls in decorator colors. They may end up dying in a corner of their cell without having really been alive for years."[11]

The lure of romance linked with dependency is a survival mechanism. It puts up a wall and keeps us from being in our own custody. The illusion works, but not very well and not for very long.

We worship romance in this culture. Even in an age of relatively easy and prevalent divorce and continued cynicism about long-term relationships, we are still a culture that likes to "fall in love." The love theme occupies many of the unfolding dramas in our Top 40 songs, daytime soap operas, prime time television and movies.

The theme is relentless: "I am somebody if I have somebody." Even our choice of language supports this illusion: "I've found the right person." Some of the illusory expectations that go along with the euphoria of romantic love include feeling completed, believing that anxieties, neuroses and traumas can be resolved, and believing that being in love will make us happy.

It's easy to understand why romance is so compelling. For when we fall in love, we are actually involved in a form of identity projection. It's our "opportunity" to move beyond the boundaries of our loneliness. Most of us experience our loneliness as painful and yearn to escape from our individual identities to unite with the world outside ourselves. By pouring ourselves into our loved one, we are, in Jungian language, making an attempt to be whole, to unite the conscious and the unconscious and get in touch with all that we are.

Falling in love happens to the best of us. In itself, it is neither wrong nor evil. In fact, it is a healthy signal of our created "bent" toward relationship and fulfillment. We get into trouble when the other person, or our "love object," becomes the entire focus of our emotional energy. We cannot do enough because our personal identity is dependent upon this "object."

Living for this "high," this romantic explosion, our relationship, or this individual, becomes secondary to our pursuit of the "right person." Consequently, says Shain, "our society isn't very big on friendship, really. We think of friends as people to spend time with when there isn't anyone else around who really matters. And sometimes when we have a vacancy for lover or spouse, we look for someone to fill that slot instead of seeing what there is, and miss what might have been."[12]

5. The fear of rejection and the need to please.

Some people's identities are so dependent upon those around them that they repress all of their own needs, wishes and desires. Decisions are made strictly on the basis of avoiding rejection or pleasing others. These individuals are like children of an alcoholic or children from a dysfunctional home who find themselves caught in a cycle of pleasing and catering to the whims of others, all the while sacrificing their own thoughts and emotions.

This addictive process called codependence is the subject of several recent books including the best seller *Women Who Love Too Much*. The logic of codependence says, "I will rescue the relationship by my sacrifice." More often than not, the sacrifice is not recognized for what it really is—a survival mechanism. There is a perpetuation of a false self and consequent difficulty in intimacy and sexuality issues. Codependence ultimately prevents us from receiving. In that light, our sexuality is short-circuited from the relational rhythms of giving and receiving to the precarious position of our needing to be the giver, rescuer, fixer, manager and nurturer.

When we are tied to this cycle, we can be tender, gentle and a great listener. You see, my identity is tied to the belief that I am somebody because I take care of someone; consequently, I take all failure personally. Sexual failure can be traumatic. I have no personal boundaries, for I believe I can control others' behaviors and I am somehow responsible for their happiness.

The irony of this "sacrificial" way of living is that instead of being selfless, our world is self-centered. For we believe we have power and control over those around us.

6. *Priggishness revisited.* Priggishness is the art of being a prig, a holier-than-thou individual who plays one-upmanship while pointing fingers and feigning innocence. One way to survive is to retreat. When we spend our energy scapegoating those around us, we posture ourselves in a comfortable place away from the real battle.

We fail to see that our posturing is, more often than not, a reaction formation—a projection of our own desires and fears on another. James Sennett says: "If certain sins are no problem for us, we cannot understand how in the world they could be a problem for anyone else. Of course, the sins with which *we* struggle are sins which require the utmost patience and understanding from our brothers and sisters (either that, or we take the easy way out by simply hiding our sins and praying that no one ever finds them out)."[13] As a means of hiding our own internal struggles, we find a scapegoat. Consciously, we may not even be aware of our projections. We may use this survival mechanism as a handy way to sprinkle others with a liberal dose of "Christianity."

How is this pattern addictive? It perpetuates a false self. Once again, we avoid our humanness—our brokenness, weakness, ordinariness and powerlessness. Like a fallen Humpty Dumpty, we see our brokenness, but quickly look away, with a desire to scurry back to the safety of the womb, retreat from life and point a finger at those who are "less" than we.

Who or what owns us? That's the real question. We come to our decision-making with an agenda. Our attempts to reduce the issue of moral choices to a behavioral problem with a list of moral and immoral actions are doomed to fail. This isn't to say there aren't behaviors that are "inherently" wrong or evil, but making moral choices isn't a behavioral issue. It's an identity issue. And it begins with me.

Our journey toward wholeness begins with an honest look at the agenda we carry. Shain points out that "love is lonely and poetic and mysterious and whether we recognize it or not, we climb into bed wrapping our identities closely around us, not knowing what we want from each other, and fearing both that it might be too much and not enough. Each of us hopes to be acknowledged, succored and validated, and waits for the other to make the first move, and if we often accept orgasm instead of what we hoped for, at some level we know the real gift is being known."[14]

It's true that most of us don't know what we want in life, but we're sure we haven't got it. It seems we're often stuck on a carrousel that doesn't stop, regardless of our good intentions. As we struggle with our addictions, we find we can't continue to ignore, repress or hide behind our correct theology or those behaviors that conceal our real self. At some point we have to face the difficult question, "To whom or what do I belong?"

▶ Discussion Questions

1. Several things can happen when we accept a behavioral view of sexuality (pages 50-53). Talk about examples of the behavioral viewpoint you see around you. Can you identify with any of the examples mentioned? Why or why not?

2. "It's who or what owns us that determines the choices we make" (pages 53-54). Do you agree or disagree? Explain. If you had to identify who or what owned you right now, could you do that? Why or why not?

3. What are the implications of living in an addictive

culture (pages 54-59)? Think about your own life. How can you relate to the dynamics in the addictive cycle?

4. The following cultural promises can become addictive and be used as survival mechanisms. How does each promise perpetuate a false image? Which promise offers the most difficult struggle for you? Explain.

Cultural Promise	How It Perpetuates a False Image
1. The performance principle (pages 59-61)	
2. A cure for loneliness (pages 61-62)	
3. The display of power (pages 62-63)	
4. The lure of romance (pages 63-64)	
5. The fear of rejection and the need to please (pages 64-65)	
6. Priggishness revisited (pages 65-66)	

► CHAPTER 4

The Trouble With Being Human

"What we look for first is not a theory of sexuality nor a set of rules for sexual behavior; we look for an understanding of what we are, what we tend to make of ourselves, and what we can be through grace."—Lewis Smedes[1]

■ ■ ■

"Life cannot be managed like pneumonia or some other disease. It demands to be understood rather than treated. We must enter into it, understanding and accepting the terms of our relationship with it, neither demanding too much nor settling for too little. And the best way to approach this is through a realistic appreciation and acceptance of what it means to be human. It is as simple and as awesome as that."—Eugene Kennedy[2]

Sexuality concerns itself with what it means to be human. That's where my discomfort begins. It means that sex and the choices I make with regard to sex cannot be divorced from Terry. There is a part of me that wants to sever my decision-making from my person. When I bring to this discussion my complex mixture of needs, illusions, addictions and belief systems, I bring my humanness—with my vulnerability, propensity to fail, fragile ego, unhealthy desires, overinflated willpower, powerlessness and wounds. Then I wonder, "Is it okay to be human?"

We all come to adulthood wounded. Each of us is a self that is alienated from its home, and we bring that woundedness to our decision-making. My fear of the incomplete— the complex, needy, human Terry—keeps me hoping to be rescued. I buy an illusion of power, an illusion that there is life without a need to be "loose and shabby in the joints," as the Velveteen Rabbit feared. Or I arrange my life around busyness, hoping to escape the grip of the inner debate with its pounding, relentless reminder of the distance between who I should be and who I really am.

Our propensity toward maintaining these illusions with regard to our identity is rooted in our belief system—the core of beliefs we have about ourselves that affect how we perceive reality. Our belief system also includes our life-long accumulation of assumptions, myths, illusions, judgments and the messages we hold to be true. In short, it's the way we perceive the world, and hence, the way we make choices in this world. The ad was right; it is "who owns us" that makes us important.

When we insist upon compartmentalizing our sexuality, we miss the point. We fail to see that our decisions are an extension of our identities. In the last two chapters we emphasized the fact that more often than not, we use sex for non-sexual needs—a need to be needed, a need to use, a need to be in control, a need to prove, and other needs. And we attempt to meet these needs with a variety of survival mechanisms such as performance, romance and codependence. In other words, the behavior itself is symptomatic of the underlying need. We cannot ignore any behavior as if it has no moral relevance, but we must realize morality is seated not in behavior, but, as Jesus reminds us, in the "heart"—the motivations or belief systems.

Our point is that sexual behavior always communicates something about our person or something about our identity. The behaviors we choose—in our minds or with our bodies—are reflections of issues and questions that make up our "identity inventory," or that which owns us. We have been so quick to collect and use arguments that will decide the scale of moral impurity for any given behavior that we, like the Levite in the parable of the good Samaritan, have left the wounded individual (who is often an arrogant and devil-may-care individual) by the side of the road, missing his or her signals of need and the call for restoration of self-worth. To understand morality, we must start with identity, self-worth and restoration of dignity.

Morality cannot be neatly compartmentalized. In the same way I need a self to be intimate, so do I also need self-esteem when I make choices. The alternative is threatening. For the "intimate" in my life becomes simply an extension of myself, and the choices I make become a reflection of my continuing search for identity.

Sam Keen explains: *"Our love proceeds more from trying to fill the hole than by allowing the whole to fill us. We become obsessed with what is missing rather than what is given . . . What we call 'love' becomes searching (in vain) for what (we imagine) we lack . . . The more we force a lover, a wife, a husband, a child, a job, a cause, a thing, or a drug to try to fill the void, the more that 'loved' one becomes a misplaced focus for eros, an idol that will inevitably disappoint us, and which we will come to hate."*[3]

My life and the choices I make become a defense against loneliness, woundedness and humanness, and our culture only reinforces the struggle. Because we have based our identities on external references, we succumb to Madison Avenue's relentless pressure to redefine who we are by what we buy. Self-esteem by consumption consistently gives way to the reality that "more is never enough." We have been inculcated with the pronouncement that we are special, with more opportunities than any other generation in the areas of career choices, relationship alternatives and financial prospects. We are caught in the crosscurrents of the times. On the one hand, we are anxious to inherit our culturally promised affluence (translated practically as immediate gratification) and the confidence that seems to explain the resurgence of the rugged American individualist. On the other hand, we are overwhelmed with what is expected. To be ordinary has become an indictment rather than a description.

We are a generation of talented, educated, bright, fast-paced young adults with more options than our parents ever dreamed of, yet we aren't comfortable with ourselves. We are not at "home." We have an address, but we cannot be found there. Our cultural context only perpetuates a "dis-eased" picture of the self—one that is never complete or at rest.

► *Sexuality and Acceptance*

To address the subject of sexuality and ethics, we must begin with acceptance. It is no coincidence that this is where the gospel begins. To experience a healthy life—and to make healthy moral choices—you need to know that you are loved, that you are worthy, that you do have dignity, that you don't need "external references." You are valuable as you are now—in all of your humanness.

To accept that reality isn't easy because it means coming face to face with ourselves. It means confession. In the last chapter we spoke of a need for honest introspection. More than just a recitation of our past or current sins, confession demands responsibility and ownership. It says, "I bring who I am today to this place, and I own who I am and what I have done with no need to justify, explain or deny." Why must we confess this reality? Because it's the first step to being at home with ourselves. The alternative is to continue to maintain the illusion that we have absolute freedom, that we are in charge of our own identities and that control is therefore of utmost importance. Living with the tyranny of this need for everyone to think well of us, we avoid coming face to face with our woundedness. We perpetuate the belief that romance, or the right performance, or controlling someone, or promiscuity or abstention for the purpose of moral finger pointing will keep the hints of our humanity and vulnerability subdued. And the addiction continues.

The cure for this addictive self lies in what Keen calls "developing the witness self." It is the knowledge that the addiction, illusion or faulty belief system cannot save me. There is no one substance, activity or person that has the capacity to satisfy me fully.[4] I need external references because I realize I am incomplete. And I am hoping that someone ("This is the one. I'm really in love this time. I just know she's the 'right' one for me!") or something ("I know it's not good for me, but you don't understand, I can't quit!") or some activity ("Oh, I never have time to get in trouble; I'm always volunteering for something at church. Do I ever have time alone? No, I wouldn't know what to do with myself!") will—consciously or subconsciously—keep me from facing that realization.

Listen again to Keen: "We find wholeness in realizing our partialness. We are saved as we recognize that we remain sinners. We arrive home when we rejoice in being on the road. We are healed when we discover that the hole in our hearts is a fertile void . . . To love is to return to a home we never left, to remember who we are."[5]

What does this mean for us? It means that only when we know we are loved in our anxiety, loneliness, restlessness, incompleteness, doubt, longing and "humanness" can we have any hope of breaking free from the tyranny of our addictive nature. In fact, it is in our humanness—our restlessness, loneliness, longing and sexuality—that we meet God, in what Pascal has called the "God-shaped vacuum" in all of us.

Understanding love and sexuality begins not with sociology, psychology, behavioral science or even religion. It begins with ontology, which is the study of being—not in isolation, but as the self is connected to other beings. We could rephrase Descartes to reflect a more accurate picture of the self: "I was loved, therefore I am."

If this is true, then I need not run from my woundedness. My delusive belief system convinces me that my identity is contingent upon my ability to prove or to perform. I must have or show some capability that will win enough merit to prove my worthiness. Under that kind of personal tyranny, I have learned to fear my shadow side—my vulnerability, weakness, loneliness and incompleteness. I have learned to orchestrate my life around the illusion that my worthiness depends upon me and how well I perform, look or act. So I rationalize my weaknesses and run from my loneliness with a full social calendar, or I adopt another person (or project) who will help me maintain my reputation as a "caretaker." I compensate for my incompleteness with a mixture of bravado and charm, and I avoid my vulnerability by maintaining a pleasant but controlled relational environment.

Where does health begin? It begins by looking at the multifaceted nature and richness—the contradictions, projections, needs, dreams and fears—of my humanity. In silence I view these personal realities with an embrace so I can hear the words of freedom, "You are loved." Keith Clark explains: "I was having a very difficult time accepting myself as I saw myself at that moment. The shallowness of my most ardent efforts became apparent. I wanted to run from it; I wanted to disengage from me! I despised myself to the point of almost becoming ill.

"I allowed my eyelids to close. Tears moistened the edges of my eyelids . . . It all felt like a sham. I wanted to be the person they (all the 'others' in his life) approved, respected, loved and appreciated. But I knew I wasn't.

"In that dark space somewhere near the core of myself, a light at first pierced and then spread. There began to dawn in that darkness the realization that God was not surprised at what I had just discovered. God had known all along! God was not having difficulty in accepting me; I was! God had accepted me in my neediness even as I was acting because of it. It was as if I had finally arrived at that hollow center of myself where God had been waiting for me, where God had been inviting me.

"I cried softly. And I wiped my eyes . . . Finally I smiled what I have always thought must be a wry sort of smile. And then it brightened into a broad smile and a laugh."[6]

I immediately recall the scene of forgiveness in the movie *The Mission*, which displays all the terror and beauty that comes with such self-revelation. A slave trader has been capturing Indians for profit and has also been accused of killing his brother. Although the law says it was self-defense, the stark realization of the extent of his selfishness has driven the slave trader to despair and self-pity. A Jesuit priest offers this man the possibility of hope and redemption. In a damp, isolated cell, the slave trader wallows in self-doubt.

"Do you know who I am?" he challenges the priest.

"Yes, you are a slave trader and a mercenary, and you killed your brother. And you loved him very much, although you chose a funny way to show it."

Undaunted in his self-hatred, the slave trader cries, "But for me, there is no redemption."

The scenes that follow play out the theme of a man in pursuit of a new identity. The slave trader accompanies the priest and other members of the Jesuit order on an arduous and dangerous trek into the South American jungles. Here the Jesuits have started a small mission where the slave trader had previously captured and killed several members of a tribe. On the journey, the man carries with him a cumbersome and heavy assortment of soldier's armor, held together by netting and attached to a strong rope that is tied to his neck and back. The load represents his penance, and the slave trader is determined to carry it to completion.

When the task appears impossible, some of the Jesuits have empathy with his burden and try to relieve the man of his bondage. But the slave trader is determined to prove something to someone—maybe to God, to the Indians or to himself.

At last the small band of missionaries arrive. As people from the tribe warmly welcome the priests, the slave trader appears some 100 yards away, slowly making his way but stooped over by the liability of his personal frailties. The Indians spot him and are silent, for they know who he is. They know it is he who has killed some of their tribe members and sold others into slavery.

Rushing forward, one of the young Indians grabs the slave trader by the hair, now matted and wet with mud and perspiration, raises the head and face for all to see, then stands poised with his hunting knife, waiting for some confirmation as to the man's fate. The slave trader's life is literally in the young Indian's hands. Time stands still. Then the decision is made. Grabbing the rope, the young tribesman uses his knife to quickly release the load the man has carried. The netting of armor plummets over the ledge, landing in the river below. With that action, the emotion pours. The slave trader begins to sob uncontrollably, and with his tears come all the guilt, sorrow and humiliation he has felt. He is free from his need to prove anything to anyone. Not understanding his sobbing, the Indians see the man's contorted, tear-streaked face and begin to laugh; soon all join in the laughter. Then as the fine line between pain and joy evaporates, the tears and laughter mingle together in a sweet symbol of reconciliation. The slave trader is invited to receive love apart from any external references. He no longer has anything to prove or to earn. No longer does he have to perform.

▶ The Invitation to Return Home

To know love is to return to a home I never left, to remember who I am. But where do I turn? Can there be reconciliation for me? Where can I go to recover my wholeness, personal harmony and proper dignity? What are my alternatives? Can those warring factions within me—the businessman and the bum, the upright "church member" and the lusting adolescent, the caring friend and the selfish cad—be integrated into who I am and can be?

I want to overlook the reality of evil—my shadow side, my capacity to use people, my capacity to be self-destructive, and my capacity to worship possessions and public opinion. I argue, as do others: "But wait, I'm a pretty good guy. Remember, this isn't my problem!" I attempt to hide behind some sexual behavioral hierarchy, pointing to what I haven't done and to the great numbers of people who have committed sins far worse than mine. And I run from my shadow side, embarrassed by the untidiness of my humanity.

I can adopt busyness or repression and work hard to bury that rich part of me that teems with desire—or even promiscuity. I may choose to live a double life, a Jekyll and Hyde existence, hoping no one discovers that I'm able to maintain the emotional fortitude for such duplicity. Yes, I can do all those things to avoid my darkness. Or I can embrace it. I can confess and own those negative parts of my existence. Like the slave trader I can use my dark side as an opportunity for creative sorrow. For once I recognize and accept my weaknesses and struggles, I can see within me an opportunity to change my mind and heart; then my dark side has the potential to produce light, love out of sorrow, life out of death.

This lesson is illumined through two parables from Anthony DeMello's book *The Song of the Bird.* [7]

> *A man who took great pride in his lawn found himself with a large crop of dandelions. He tried every method he knew to get rid of them. Still they plagued him.*
>
> *Finally he wrote the Department of Agriculture. He enumerated all the things he had tried and closed his letter with the question: "What shall I do now?"*
>
> *In due course the reply came: "We suggest you learn to love them."*

The second parable reads as follows:

> *He was becoming blind by degrees. He fought it with every means in his power. When medicine no longer served to fight it, he fought it with his emotions. It took courage to say to him, "I suggest you learn to love your blindness."*
>
> *It was a struggle. He refused to have anything to do with it in the beginning. And when he eventually brought himself to speak to his blindness his words were bitter. But he kept on speaking*

*and the words slowly changed into words of res-
ignation and tolerance and acceptance . . . and,
one day, very much to his own surprise, they became words of friendliness . . . and love. Then
came the day when he was able to put his arm
around his blindness and say, "I love you." That
was the day I saw him smile again.*

*His vision, of course, was lost forever. But
how attractive his face became!*

In the same way, once I experienced confession and acceptance, I lost my ability to be in control forever. But oh,
how light my burden became. My need to be powerful was
lost forever, but how welcome the gift of life became. My
hard-fought task of staying above the struggle of my sexuality was lost forever, but how freeing it was to give up the
tension of living life as a great pretender.

In confession, we no longer need to bury our neediness
or desire. Along with St. Augustine we can sigh that we are
weary at last and can finally give up our battle to defend
our reputation (that mountain of which we were the self-
proclaimed monarch) and our need for absolute freedom.
We can with all others who have gone through The Twelve
Steps program of Alcoholics Anonymous confess that we
"are powerless," for we realize lives are built on a foundation of neediness. Life can now be a gift. We no longer
need to take it, earn it or deserve it.

Powerless and needy—doesn't such a view depress people? It does if we assume that powerless equals worthless.
Only in confession are we ultimately free. For our identity
is intact in the hands of a loving, faithful Creator, not in our
accomplishments or expertise; not in our goodness or
screw ups; and not in who we know, where we've been or
what we haven't done. Our identity resides only in a Creator who doesn't quit on us. Only then can we afford
intimacy, for no longer do we have to prove anything.

It's difficult to accept this concept because we're not
used to having people love us just because they want to
love us. We're used to trying to measure up, only to come
up short. We're used to opening up to love, only to be be-

trayed. We're used to keeping our noses clean for credit, only to realize there's no payoff for such moral innocence.

Before sexuality and the choices we make can be behavioral issues, they must first be faith issues. But "the question is not whether we believe in [God], but whether He believes in us. And we have the absolute promise—the Flesh of His Son—that He does. God is the Faithful One. He is faithful even to us."[8]

God's infinite love and our human dignity in the face of that love set the course for whatever we do with regard to theology, rules and ethical mandates. For in the face of that love, "no one is to be treated as an it. All people are to be treated as God treats us. This is the touchstone. We become followers of Jesus as we love other people with the same kind of self-giving, unjudging love as he gives us."[9]

There is, of course, a lot more ground to cover before this book is complete. But any look at theology, biblical foundations, decision-making filters or community building would miss the point without the essential reality of knowing that our identity is intact in the hands of a loving and faithful God. It doesn't matter how sophisticated we may be with regard to sexuality—how scared, how anxious or how morally pure. The point is simple. Because we are loved, we don't have to prove anything to anyone. That means that our sexuality need not be an arena for identity performance. Nor does our morality need to be a platform from which we prove to the world how righteous we really are. Nor are we forever chained to relentless self-defeating patterns of behavior that manipulate and use both ourselves and those around us. In the face of the gospel, our agenda is no longer determined by a world that measures life in terms of productivity quotas. We begin with acceptance, and here is the good news, my friends: "When we were still powerless . . . God [demonstrated] his own love for us in this: While we were still sinners, Christ died for us" (Romans 5:6, 8).

▶ Discussion Questions

1. What does it mean to "come to adulthood wounded"

(page 70)? How does our belief system perpetuate our woundedness?

2. "To understand morality, we must start with identity, self-worth and restoration of dignity" (page 71). Explain what this statement means to you and how you would use it to define morality for yourself. Talk about the parts that acceptance and confession play in coming to terms with your sexuality.

3. Reread the story of Keith Clark (pages 74-75) and the story from *The Mission* (pages 75-76). How do these two stories compare? What is the significance of the tears turning to laughter at the end of both stories? What do these stories say to you?

4. What does it mean to "learn to love your dandelions" (page 77)? Think of your own "dandelions" you must learn to love. Which ones offer the greatest challenge for you?

5. The question is not whether we believe in God, but whether he believes in us (page 79). How do we know what God believes about us?

►SECTION TWO:

Biblical Foundation

Introduction

*T*here are no casual discussions about sex. Just beneath the surface they are accompanied by unasked questions, self-doubt, comparison, irrational urges, conflicting needs and a hope for emotional freedom. Our attempts to theologize about our sexuality can be a convenient way of distancing ourselves from the real battlefield within our own hearts and minds. If we know the right answers, we convince ourselves that relationships will go smoother, conflict will be erased and we can view life from the vantage point of our "having arrived"—as if life is lived on the basis of responses to a multiple-choice test.

Can our theology touch who we are—our emotions, needs, laughter, raw edges and tears? In an already emotionally charged arena, now is the time for us to use our ability to think to build a personally satisfying moral attitude. Too often, we use the Bible as a club. We look shocked, we moralize, we sermonize, we condemn, we impose. Now isn't the time for another variation of the easy-to-market, shock-value theology. More than ever we need clear thinking.

As a Christian, I believe the Bible is God's Word regarding human life and morals. We need permission not to hide behind our fears (including our sexuality) or our inadequate pictures of God and the world. If God does speak, we need permission to hear what is said so we are not left in an ethical vacuum.

Section Two examines our theology. Our purpose is not to impose, but to examine what we have assumed to be ethical imperatives, to separate the wheat from the chaff, the valid from the invalid, and to create a logical and coherent moral theology.

So let's think together. Don't be afraid to ask questions, doubt, disagree or learn. And above all, remember that our purpose with theology is not to hide, but to reveal.

CHAPTER 5

Created as Body-Persons

"We have been wonderfully and beautifully made and we need to have a total vision of life in which love and salvation permeate every area of our lives—including our sexuality."—Morton Kelsey[1]

When asked why he became a Christian, an experienced naturalist and mountain climber responded: "Convergence. In the same way that the world below converges when I observe it from the top of a mountain peak. In the same way that the world is more celebrative when I see the big picture. That's what my faith does for me."

That's what we need to deal with in the issue of our sexuality—convergence. We must have the ability to see our sexuality and the choices we make in a larger context than that of our own inhibitions, projections, desires and genitals. We need to see how our choices are not and cannot be compartmentalized and dismissed as whim or irrelevant. We need to comprehend the unfolding of belief systems and the personal wars we wage to protect the illusions we carry to prevent life from hurting us. We need to see that ethics is relational, that our choices cannot be seen apart from the world in which we live and that they do in fact impact who we become.

Or, are we on our own on this one? Are there any clues, signals, rules, commands, alarms, precedents or guides? Has God spoken, and if he has, can we understand what was said in the culture in which we live? Does what God has to say make sense in the '80s and '90s in our post-Freud and post-pill America? Are the rules the same for every generation, or have they changed from our parents' time?

In the previous chapter, we found that ethics begins with a statement of faith, and so does our theology of life. We begin with the reality of a personal Creator who continues in relationship with and expresses personal concern over his creation. In the beginning was relationship; consequently, we are not left to our own devices and ingenuity to make life work. There is a context for the development of human relationships, the expression of human values and the maturation of life itself. Nothing can be more healing than sensing the religious significance of our lives and the mysteries of life we experience because of how we were created.

Our temptation, however, is not toward convergence, but toward control. We do not want an invitation to life; we want to overcome it. That's why we are tempted to turn immediately to the didactic portions of the Bible. We want to reduce life's mysteries to a verse which creates the illusion that the issue is resolved simply because we have pronounced a verdict. Just as total chaos (or universal personal whim) is one extreme, so is total control (or order) the other extreme, a world where mystery is eliminated and responsible human freedom is diminished because of fear.

How do we begin to think clearly about the issues of sexuality and choices? That's the task before us, and it's no easy job for two reasons. One, there is no shortage of available material detailing the discussions about human sexuality, and we hardly intend to resolve the debate in this writing. In recent years, there has been much helpful psychological information to supplement the observations made here. Perhaps an openness to this continuing dialogue may encourage progressive development and growth.

Two, we all come to this task with a variety of old wives' tales, inadequate information and misconceptions. In Chapter 2, we looked at some of our myths and misconceptions. We need to be reminded of these as we continue to unfold a clear way of thinking and theologizing about sexuality and ethics.

Where do we turn for this convergence? Does the Bible speak? Is there a Christian way of thinking? Is it understandable? The answer to these three questions is yes, and it will be our task in the next two chapters to unfold the central themes of a Christian way of thinking. These themes are not contained in a random, proof-text approach to the Bible, so it will not do for us to merely cite chapter and verse. We need to step back—as did our mountain-climbing friend—and see the bigger picture of what the Bible communicates. We need to stop and listen to the heartbeat of the gospel—the culmination of God's revelation through the Incarnate Word, Jesus Christ. Let's look at four biblical themes that talk about who we are and what we intend to make of ourselves. We'll cover the first two themes in this chapter and the last two in Chapter 6.

1. God is life-giving. Too often we ask what God says before we ask who he is. Our preconceived notions about God can predetermine the way we build our theological frameworks. Our ideas about God come from a variety of places—parents, church, friends and the culture in which we live. Too often we accept particular perceptions without weighing their merit or implications. When it comes to our sexuality, for instance, most of us picture God as "someone who is on the other team."

We assume God is the angry judge, the capricious Creator, the displeased parent or, at best, the disinterested deity. In my conversations with young adults, God is pictured as far away, displeased, irritated and toying with his creation.

When we perceive God's presence as conditional, we encourage the attitude of performance for worth as it's promoted in our culture.

Such a distortion of God is guaranteed to distort the way we view God's creation, which includes our bodies and the way we understand love and human relationships. Our values and moral choices become predicated on a theological foundation—conscious or subconscious—that is built on fear.

In contrast, our human dignity statements in Chapter 4 are predicated on a theological foundation that says our God is a God of love. We believe the God we actively worship seeks and intends our best interest; he wants us healthy, fully alive and whole. Our God is life-giving. How do we know this to be true? How do we come to know God? We come to know him by looking at what he does—or has done. In Jesus, God is made flesh. Within this person, God acts in history, time and flesh. In the incarnation we see that this God "was an incredibly loving parent with many of the best qualities of mother and father. Abba cared for us all, good and bad, and made the sun to rise on the good and the evil, on the just and the unjust, on those who follow the sexual laws and those who deviate from them. Like the father of the prodigal this Divine Lover is not interested in punishing those who mess up their lives but in offering new possibilities and opportunities."[2]

There is something in all of us that wants to begin with a theology of a life-giving God and then immediately amend whatever we say with a sentence that begins with "But," "If" or "When." That kind of thinking portrays a concept of God that involves a reciprocal payoff or a mandated performance. Andrew Greeley explains: "Whether premarital or extramarital sex is sinful is not nearly so important as whether Christianity can sustain the positive demands of faithfulness. If it can, then the question of sex outside of marriage can be answered within a religious context. If it cannot, then the church is simply one more ethical or moral lawgiver with nothing new or unique to add to human customs. The reason why we Christians are faithful in our relationships to one another is that Yahweh is faithful to us."[3] The context of our identity—secure in the hands of a faithful God—forms the foundation for our life-giving ethical system.

Translation? We serve a God who will not quit on us. We may turn our backs, but he won't. He has made it perfectly clear, from Genesis to Revelation, that no matter what his people do, he will not turn his back. So when God speaks about our ethical well-being, he speaks as our advocate, not as our enemy.

2. God created us as body-persons. "In the very beginning," writes Mel White, "God had a wonderful sexual fantasy . . . Sex has been a part of God's dream for us from the beginning. He didn't snicker or giggle or gasp and turn away when Adam and Eve presented themselves naked for His final clearance check."[4] The biblical record is clear: God created sex. And it's important to remind ourselves that we aren't simply dealing with what we do with our genitals. (Such thinking reduces the entire issue of sexual morality to intercourse.) For when we say that God created sex, we mean precisely what Genesis tells us: "The Lord God formed the man from the dust of the ground and breathed into his nostrils the breath of life, and the man became a living being" (Genesis 2:7). "So God created man in his own image . . . male and female he created them" (Genesis 1:27).

Who we are as people is intricately interwoven with who we are as bodies. We are "spirit-enlivened" bodies, or in Lewis Smedes' phrase, "body-persons." We don't just carry a body around; we are a body. Our "bodyness" includes our maleness and femaleness; our need for human touch; our attractions; our hormones; our pleasures of smell, taste, sight and touch; our capacity for longing and loneliness; and our restlessness for completion in another. Our bodyness cannot be severed from who we are personally and spiritually.

It was theologian Karl Barth who challenged our modern confinement of the image of God in man. It is not accidental or incidental that we were created male and female—sexual body-persons. In fact, says Barth, it is our sexuality that is the Godlike image in us, the "imago-dei." Our sexuality, then, is the center of our humanity.

While many theologians argue about this exact point of reference (God's image in us), it is not our task to resolve the complexities of this debate. We merely need to remind ourselves of the profound impact our sexuality has on our spiritual identity as creations in the image of God. And lest we forget, we refer here not only to the list of genital and pregenital behaviors, but to the full and mysterious range of what it means to be human and fully alive as a body.

For it is our sexual nature that reminds us both of our uniqueness as individuals—male and female—and of our need for communion. Our humanness and sexuality reflect the reality that we are not self-contained units, capable of existing in a vacuum. We are by our created nature compelled into relationships. With more than just the hormonal urge toward physical intercourse, we recognize the full range of our humanity—and therefore our sexuality—that sees life in relationship: in touching, caring, trusting, listening, needing, embracing and loving. Individuals are created in God's image, but they represent God's image only when they personally relate to others in a loving relationship—not only marriage, but the human relationship.

My ability to make good, healthy decisions about my body is predicated on a good, healthy understanding about my being a body-person. Yes, I am a part of a generation that prides itself in its liberal attitudes toward nudity and public physical expression, a generation that has given birth to the casual and chatty approach to sexual dynamics, a generation whose sophistication seems to far surpass earlier Victorian generations of our parents and grandparents. Yet, have I—or have we—learned to be at home with our bodies? Have we learned how to fully embrace what it means to be a body-person? Does our continued reluctance to discuss physical and sexual issues impact the way we make decisions?

If we do not come to terms with our creation as body-persons, we often drift—sometimes consciously, mostly subconsciously—between two unhealthy extremes: The body is sinful or the body is inconsequential.

The body is sinful. This extreme chooses to separate our bodies from our person. It's nothing new. Centuries of people, including our modern world, have lived with this dichotomy, this split in which the spirit is perceived as good and the body is perceived as evil. This concept has served Christianity well—especially in recent times when there has been an emphasis on the behaviorist approach to our identity in an attempt to create a regimented and disciplined code of morality.

Where did this dichotomy originate? Certainly not from the Hebrew writers, who throughout the Old Testament present us with an earthy, matter-of-fact picture of human sexuality. In their book *Sacrament of Sexuality*, Morton Kelsey and Barbara Kelsey contend that the culprit was Gnosticism. The gnostic attitude of creation came out of Persian thinking in which there were "two equal and opposite divine creative forces—the light and the dark . . . Matter was seen as ugly, recalcitrant, irredeemable and evil. The creation of human beings . . . was an imprisoning of pure and holy spirit in vile matter." The only way to achieve salvation was by eliminating any attachment to the world of physical reality and by getting rid of emotional involvement and physical pleasure. At times this thinking was carried to the extreme when it taught that bringing children into the world was ultimately evil, in fact, "anything to do with conception or copulation or sexuality or genital organs was evil or ugly."[5]

We can trace most of the influence for this thinking to St. Augustine of Hippo (A.D. 354-430). For nine years prior to his conversion, Augustine was a member of a gnostic sect that held a religious philosophy known as Manichaeism. The influence of that view of reality impacted his teaching on sexuality and has ultimately influenced the way we think today. Kelsey writes that Augustine went so far as to say "even normal sexual intercourse within marriage can be venial sin; the quicker married people abstain from all sexual relations the better for their souls. For Augustine all sexual acts or pleasure outside of marriage were mortal sins—acts sufficient to separate people forever from God and so consign them to hell."[6]

I was raised in this dichotomy of reality. And subconsciously, I began to distrust all physical pleasure. I approached life as if there had to be a choice between that which was physical and that which was spiritual. I was constantly reminded that Christians do not think "those things" or at least let anyone know they are thinking them. I was also cautioned not to feel those things or give in to those indulgences. I was warned not to enjoy life to any extreme and was continually reminded that the "heathens" weren't really having fun anyway.

So what was I to do? On the one hand, I wanted to be a "good Christian"—spiritual, righteous and holy (not realizing, of course, that I still perceived spirituality as only something I did). On the other hand, I was fully aware of my desire to be "physical"—I wanted to be needed, touched, longed for and craved by another. It seemed as if my holiness and my horniness were to be mutually exclusive, and my task was to constantly fight the difficult choice between these two alternatives, one for God and the other for the flesh. To live this way, I had no alternative but to repress anything that hinted of my sexuality.

But repression is denial. It's like living as if a part of me doesn't exist. Psychiatrists have likened it to attempting to keep a large beach ball under water. In reality, of course, I cannot do so without having both of my hands occupied. Thus, I am no longer free to function at full capacity. The same is true with repression of my emotions, feelings and desires. Once the beach ball is released, it explodes to the surface, much like my repressed sexuality, out of control and working itself out in ways that are unhealthy and inappropriate.

The irony is that kind of repression takes a lot of energy and only ensures us that our attention stays focused on what we are attempting to deny. In psychological terms, that which we repress owns us. It determines our identity. And it's no coincidence that repressed sexuality finds a way to express itself in projection, moralizing, voyeurism, sermonizing, judgmentalism, anger and addictive personalities.

I had never been given permission to be thankful for

who I am as a body-person—to thank God for my need for human companionship, my need to be touched, my excitement in watching an attractive woman walk by, my loneliness when I feel isolated, my fascination and curiosity with my own body. Instead, I've learned to view my physical needs and pleasure with contempt, played out in a continual but personal love-hate war. My repression has become the means for me to buy my spirituality—a spirituality which, unfortunately, was not ulcer-free.

The body is inconsequential. The other extreme in this spirit-body dualism says that what I do with my body doesn't really matter. It has no impact on who I am as a spiritual being. What I do with my genitals has no bearing on my spiritual life. When we understand this extreme, we can see that our cultural tendency toward pornography is not a swing toward a more progressive view of sexuality, but a reinforcement of this same dualism. By placing emphasis upon the genitals (as most pornographic magazines and films do), sex is trivialized. The physical body is ripped from the context of the whole person and becomes simply an instrument or an object for generating pleasure. Recognizing our creation as body-persons prohibits this continual ripping, or personal destruction, that divides our humanness.

To say the body is inconsequential is to believe the body can somehow be divorced from human relationship. A prostitute was asked in an interview how she could do what she did night after night. She answered: "Oh, you need to understand. It's not me in that room, it's just my body." Such a gift of one's body cannot be offered without tearing at or severing the emotions. We begin to lose touch with other feelings such as celebration, mystery and awe.

Ron Nicholl reminds us: "What we do with our bodies, what we put into them, how we treat them, what use we make of them, these are spiritual tasks which we are called to carry out in the name of holiness. There is no division in reality between the material and the spiritual; our spirituality is manifested by our treatment of matter."[7]

Take a look at the two extremes in the chart on the following page.

An Inadequate Theology:
The World Is a Dualism

The body is sinful.	The body is inconsequential.
The physical world: • includes "all that which is evil." • encourages you to ignore your spiritual nature.	**The spiritual world:** • includes "all that which is good." • says the physical doesn't matter.

Two extremes. In one, the church tells us to repress our physical nature. In the other, our culture tells us to ignore our related spiritual nature. Both positions are dangerous and both are built on an inadequate theology that says the world is a dualism. It's not uncommon for us to fluctuate back and forth between these two extremes, periodically putting our spiritual self on the shelf while we are driven to act out in some area of sexual expression. The result is a Jekyll and Hyde drama, in which the individual pays a heavy emotional price for his or her inability to own the full range of what it means to be human. The "emotional payment" is extracted not for the acting out, but for our inability to integrate all of life.

Harold Kushner comments on that ongoing drama: "We have inherited both the Greek love of physical pleasure and the biblical ambivalence about it. We are torn between finding physical pleasures irresistible and finding them shameful and guilt-producing . . . We cannot possibly be content if we are constantly at war with ourselves, if our bodies and our consciences are engaged in perpetual struggle, one calling the other a pervert and the other responding by shouting back, 'Prude!' . . . How can we even approach inner peace and contentment when one half of us hates and scorns our other half?"[8]

Reading Genesis should invoke a sense of celebration within us. It offers an invitation to embrace the okayness of who we are as fully human and fully sexual. It further inspires a sense of reverence for the mystery of human relationships and sexual dynamics.

Smedes observes that "body-persons have a side to them that is wildly irrational, splendidly spontaneous and beautifully sensuous. This is not a regrettable remnant of the beast in human beings, a fiendish enemy in man's personal cold war within himself. It is a gift that comes along with being body-persons. Some Christians may wish that God had stuck with making angels; but God was delighted to have body-persons."9

Our need for a sense of reverence was brought to my attention by a friend. I had just shared with him my frustration over a seemingly constant preoccupation with staring at women's bodies while at the beach. He smiled and then suggested, "Why don't you just thank God for your ability to appreciate what you see?" No doubt I looked surprised—primarily because I had never pictured God as part of anything that had to do with my sexuality.

My friend went on. "When you thank God, three things take place. First, you acknowledge the reality that you and your body, including your thoughts, feelings and desires, were created by him. Second, you bring your feelings and desires to the conscious level—only there can you deal with them, only there can you make choices. Your only other alternative is repression, and you've been trying that. Obviously it's not working, for you are more preoccupied now than ever before. Third, you acknowledge—if not consciously, then subconsciously—who owns that body you are enjoying with your eyes. You realize it is not an object for use or abuse. Now you can make behavioral choices, not out of compulsion or fear, but out of responsibility."

What makes us assume we must act out any and every feeling we enjoy or experience? Sometimes I don't want physical enjoyment or experience; I want to idolize. For example, when two friends touch in the elevator and feel a brief spark between them, they are experiencing a touch of divine unity. It would seem that for these two people "the proper reaction is neither to find a bedroom where they can have quick intercourse nor to be deeply chagrined at the power of their own passions; rather, I think, they should be grateful for the spark of the divine that is present in them and the revelation, however briefly, of the power of that spark."10

Any discomfort I might feel from being told that my

sexuality sparks a reflection of the divine—of God's handi-work—is related to the continuing war I wage with my body. For my body takes turns being an enemy I must sub-due (or at best a child I need to retrain) or being a disposable house I inhabit as I pass through this life to a better and more spiritual life.

There's a striking remark found in the Talmud (the books of Jewish wisdom) that says in the world to come, each of us will be called to account for all the good things God put on Earth which we refused to enjoy. It's the kind of statement we wouldn't want to make without a disclaim-er, but, says Kushner, in this statement there is "no scorn, no disgust for the body and its appetites. Instead, a sense of reverence for the pleasures of life which God put here for our enjoyment, a way of seeing God in the world through the experience of pleasant moments. Like all gifts, of course, they can be misused, but then the fault is ours, not God's . . . Used properly, all of these appetites come to be seen as God's gifts to us, to add pleasure to our lives."[11]

And God said, "It is good." It is user-friendly! This body—our body—with all its drives, needs, desires, urges, appetites, passions, contradictions and emotions—is good! Although we want to fully understand and perhaps in that way gain some control over this wild and unpredictable na-ture of ours, it's hard to say the only two words God wishes us to say: "Thank you." Maybe we just need to stop and let the words from the creation narrative in Genesis sink in. "It is good." Our body is not a problem to solve, or an enigma to untangle, but a mystery and a gift to be celebrated.

► Discussion Questions

1. Is it possible to seek "convergence" in the area of our sexuality without needing closure (pages 85-87)? (Or how can we examine the choices we make in a larger con-text than our own needs and desires?)

2. What does it mean to you that God is life-giving (pag-es 87-89)? How do you picture God in relation to your sexuality? How does this image influence your thoughts and feelings about your relationship with God?

3. What does it mean to you that God created you as a body-person (pages 89-90)?

4. How do you relate to the dualism of the spirit and the body—the spirit as good and the body as evil (page 91)? What happens when we choose to repress, reject or ignore the physical? How has this dualism affected you personally?

5. How can we celebrate and be thankful for our bodies and our sexuality? Think about your own sexuality. What do you like most about being male or female? You may wish to list qualities you appreciate and celebrate each quality in a special way.

►CHAPTER 6

Commandments That Fit

"There is a 'strain toward permanence' in sexual relationships."—Andrew Greeley[1]

We were created as body-persons. We may wish it to be different, or less complicated, but the fact remains, we are body-persons. Consequently, our sexuality—who we are as body-persons and what we do with our bodies—is personal. It cannot be stripped from a personal and therefore spiritual context. My choices affect me personally, and they affect you personally. Our choices are by nature relationally invested in that they are inextricably woven into who we are. Sex is not just about right and wrong behaviors, or perfecting techniques for pleasure or genital play. Sex is about who I am as a person—a body-person—and who you are as a person, and what we make of ourselves and one another in our relationship as body-persons.

Our theology of sexuality and moral choices—which we began to look at in Chapter 5—begins with a statement about God, not about us. We were created in the image of a relational God and invited by that same God to enjoy life—

with him and with one another—in a relational and physical context. His incarnation through Jesus Christ confirms
the holiness of our physical context. As body-persons we
are invited to celebrate life and wholeness. Unfortunately,
our inadequate perceptions of God distort our views of our
bodies, the purpose of morality and healthy choice-making
and, consequently, the purpose of life itself.

Our sexuality is both mysterious and powerful. There is
something in all of us that wishes to reduce our sexuality to
an understandable set of propositions, a predictable area of
human weakness and need, a lapse in willpower and resur-
facing of our old nature, or at worst, a containable inconvenience. We wish for some way to make the issue easier to handle, some guarantee that would alleviate our fear over whether
these issues will plague us forever. So we hide behind our
busyness, sophistication, rules (those illusions we use as
protective badges of purity) and continue moralizing about
those who are less spiritual than we are. We hope that no one
can see what we are really like. We also hope that our busyness, sophistication and rules will provide us with the necessary relief from sexual pressure.

We feel trapped. On the one hand, we find it difficult to
define or control our desires, urges, emotions and fantasies.
On the other hand, we are afraid that if there are any rules
to govern this area of our lives, they will be handed down
by a "kill-joy" God as a means of dampening our freedom.

Does this God—this life-giving, personally involved,
personally invested God—speak about our ethical condition? If this is a play with a plot and there are no open
ends, where do we turn to hear him speak? Is the Bible relevant to our lives in this age of educational sophistication?
Our questions lead us to the third biblical theme that will
continue to help us clarify our thinking.

3. God's commandments fit life's design. Our bodies and sexual feelings were created to be user-friendly. The
same can be said for God's commands—his personal statements regarding the ethical and relational well-being of his
creation. They too are user-friendly. God isn't trying to
trick us, throw us a curve or communicate in code. When

God speaks, he does so in a personal, historical and concrete way. He is more than a disinterested cosmic bystander; he is above all else a relational God. And as such, we find his communication with his people in many areas other than the recorded "Thou shalts" or "Thou shalt nots." He speaks to us in the cries of the poor and the outcasts, through trauma and tragedy, through incarnation and even through silence.

But we don't want user-friendly; we want closure. We want to be able to turn to a certain part of the Bible and find a few verses that cover every detail of life's complex decisions. If all the specifications aren't there, we make them up and insert them. And if a rule doesn't fit our situation exactly, we knock off the bothersome rough spots of reality just enough to make the situation fit our rule. When we fail to trust the giver of the law as gracious and relational, we become dependent upon the law or the rules for our identity. Then our need for closure becomes even more important.

Are we saying that God speaks? Yes. Does that mean he provides us a handbook for every detail of human behavior? No. God is concerned about the life of his creation. In that concern, he speaks—not about every nuance of life, but about life, relationships and choices that include sex and our bodies. God knows that because we are created in his image, we desire a full life and healthy relationships. But we also want to be in control, and we want not just contingent freedom, but absolute freedom.

Our desire for control has led us to idolatry. We seek fullness of life—salvation, redemption and wholeness—in finite things such as money, wealth, power, happiness, sex, prestige and our reputation. As a result we are broken people. We are addicted to our own sinfulness and our shortsightedness. In this context, God speaks. We have all violated our bent toward fullness of life. We've rejected the image in which we were created and done some pretty bad things. We've loved things and used people.

Without a healthy picture of God, it's easy to look at his actions as arbitrary and even capricious. It's as if God created the Ten Commandments as a direct result of his boredom—as if one day he had nothing especially important to occupy his time, so he took note of all the things that humans particularly enjoyed and wrote some commandments prohibiting such behavior. In reality, we see that this is not true. We are created as life-producing creatures—life-giving creations who are by our nature defined and confined by life-producing, or life-giving, parameters.

We have misunderstood God's interest in our ethical well-being, and our misunderstandings are reflected in our theology of sin—our brokenness. For in our behavioral mind-set, we too often see sin as simply an accumulation of specific behaviors that some moral code has determined as wrong or against God. "Sin! Modern man hates the word, jokes about it, wishes it away. We think that God is the cause of our inconvenience, that He has cut off the good and exciting things. We forget that something is not evil *because* God called it sin. God has called it sin, because it *is* evil, destructive to His dream for us, a death trap. God loves us too much to leave those trails unmarked."[2]

When we hear Lewis Smedes' assurance that God's commands fit life's design, we shouldn't be surprised. For God's laws merely tell us to do what we already know we should do.[3] This is really the argument of Paul, who says in the book of Romans: "(Indeed, when Gentiles, who do not have the law, do by nature things required by the law, they are a law for themselves, even though they do not have the law, since they show that the requirements of the law are written on their hearts, their consciences also bearing witness, and their thoughts now accusing, now even defending them.) This will take place on the day when God will judge men's secrets through Jesus Christ, as my gospel declares" (Romans 2:14-16). Such statements about morality hardly guarantee that people will do what they "know to do." We've already alluded to our addictive nature and our drive for control and absolute freedom. Because of these personal needs, we make moral choices that go against the nature of our creation.*

---

*Not all rules, of course, are moral rules—that is, rules about what it means to be human and loving and just. There are also rules of etiquette and rules of culture. But concern over these categories is not within the realm of this book.

But the problem is with *us*, not with moral law. Moral law fits because people were created to do the things moral law commands. Frederick Buechner simplifies this idea with the following explanation: "In order to be healthy, there are certain rules you can break only at your peril . . . Avoid bottles marked poison, don't jump out of boats unless you can swim, etc. In order to be happy, there are also certain rules you can break only at your peril . . . Get rid of hatred and envy, tell the truth, avoid temptations to evil you're not strong enough to resist, don't murder, steal, etc. . . . Both sets of rules . . . describe not the way people feel life ought to be but the way they have found life is."[4]

Moral rules are predicated by the parameters of life itself. They are ingrained in the fabric of creation—and into what it means to be human. The call for human rights is not just a good idea or a religious mandate or a majority vote. It is the inevitable outcry whenever human dignity is violated. Smedes states it this way: " 'Thou shalt' can be translated 'Everyone ought.' What must be obeyed because of God's authority ought also to be obeyed because what he commands matches what we are and what we are meant to be. The commander is the Creator; what he expects all of us to do fits what he created us to be."[5] God's speaking is inevitably in line with his creation.

But what about the specific issue of sexuality? Does the Bible speak in a specific way? How do its words match who we are?

The Bible, sex and commitment. Ironically, the Bible says little about sex. There is no embarrassment about human sexuality and earthiness, especially throughout the Old Testament. It seems the biblical writers were primarily concerned with the issues of human justice and the outworking of love. But it is in that same context that the Bible gives us a framework for understanding genital sexual behavior. Because our sexuality is tied to who we are, when we give ourselves genitally, we give all of ourselves. Consequently, sexual expression becomes an issue of justice and love. Because we are body-persons, sex (or what we do with our bodies) has a context; it can never be an end in itself. Sex is, in essence, relational and spiritual and is related to personal and spiritual growth.

Genital sex can be used as a weapon, a tool for manipulation, a cruel tease, or it can be used as a powerful affirmation of love and grace or a healing and loving balm. Why? George Leonard (who in the '60s was the leading proponent for the "free sex" movement and has in the '80s changed his mind) answers: "When I join your body, I participate in all joining. I join all of me with all of you . . . We join in full awareness, fully responsible, willing to endure times of separation and waiting, false starts, aimless play, foolishness, vulnerability, strenuous effort, total surrender. In that joining is ecstasy and sadness (it can't last forever; it must end) and also transformation: the creation of a new whole greater than the sum of its parts, an opening to deeper mysteries."[6]

It's no wonder, then, that the Apostle Paul talks seriously about the man who "unites himself with a prostitute," and argues that he becomes "one with her in body" (1 Corinthians 6:16). This is not just a behavioral issue; it is an ontological, or being, issue. Certain behaviors affront who we are. They violate our humanness by being unfair, unjust, hurtful or self-indulgent.

In light of our urge to moralize out of either guilt or projection, we need to remember that sexual intercourse doesn't join two people unless they choose to be joined. Even though this physical action has a spiritual significance, the act is immoral unless both people accept its deeper significance in their lives. For if we are body-persons, we speak not only with our voice but with our bodies. Books on what has been called body language refer to gestures, facial expressions and body posturing, but we can carry the concept even further to include the body language we speak as genital beings—as body-persons.

The Bible's concern over the context of genital sexual behavior in a sustained and committed relationship is therefore not surprising. A popular comedian used to remark, "Are you writing a check with your mouth that your body can't cash?" We can also wonder, "Are we writing checks with our bodies that our emotions can't cash?" Unless we express our sexual behaviors in a context of commitment, the behaviors will have little meaning. Without trust and fidelity, there is no way two people will develop a growing relationship. Without commitment, there is no framework on which to base behavior.

Keith Clark explains the dynamic involved. "Genital behavior does more than suggest something; it *promises*. I may not intend that meaning when I engage in intercourse with another, but I cannot escape the meaning implied in the behavior . . . If enough of us engage in genital sexual behavior and do not intend to be there for each other in the future, we all suffer because we all are losing the meaning that the behavior has in itself. Intercourse for recreation without a commitment . . . is not *human* sexuality."[7]

Why? As part of our sexuality, we are created with a capacity for intimacy—trust, connectedness and commitment—and our capacity to culminate such promises with our bodies is a freedom we want to protect. "Orgasms are nice, but affection and tenderness are indispensable. A lover does indeed provide delight, but he also protects, provides care, and helps to avoid discouragement, weariness, and boredom."[8] So what's at stake if we don't recognize the intimate part of our sexuality? We may lose the people, relationships and fragile bonds we have created out of our mutual trust and commitment.

The issue of sexuality is hardly resolved. Many questions remain unanswered. We've spoken here primarily about genital behavior. But what about pregenital behavior? What about masturbation, lust, petting, mutual masturbation, fetishes, emotional "affairs," oral sex, and the use of vibrators and contraceptives? And what about homosexual behavior? Where do we begin to develop a theology to cover the whole range of sexual involvement?

Like the religious leaders of Jesus' time, we want a full-range behavioral manual with complete specifications. We want a theology that offers closure. Jesus didn't oblige the leaders of the past nor does he oblige us. He sounds encouraging when he clearly proclaims, "I have not come to abolish the [Law or the Prophets] but to fulfill them" (Matthew 5:17). But he clarifies his statement by explaining that the law is summed up in the law of love. He reminds us to "love the Lord your God with all your heart and with all your soul and with all your mind and with all your strength" and to "love your neighbor as yourself" (Mark 12:30-31).

Jesus gave a radical new emphasis to the law. No longer was the law an oppressive tyrant, measuring every nuance of human behavior in order to determine human worth and pronounce the inevitable judgment. In the new law Jesus gave us permission to love, permission to build community, permission to say yes to our promises, commitments and relationships. He also gave us permission to say yes to human dignity and yes to loving people instead of things. "Love turns the negative 'Don'ts' into positive 'Do's.' Love turns the passive avoidance of evil into the active doing of good. Love translates the morality of 'live and let live' into a morality of 'love and help others live.' Law without love tells us not to kill a stranger; law with love moves us to go out of our way to help a wounded enemy."9

The biblical record doesn't provide us with a convenient rule book on how to win divine approval. Instead, it points us to Jesus, the incarnational fulfillment of the God who relentlessly pursues his creation to give fullness of life. This God seeks to provide his creation with a change of heart, so that we will value what's commanded rather than what's forbidden. This Christian ethic will offer us wholeness and an invitation to moral living, not necessarily a rule book completely free from ambiguity or the gray shades of life. This foundation will lead us to the fourth biblical theme that will help us clarify our sexuality.

4. Only life-giving behaviors are morally right. Our questions to God about certain behaviors are in turn his questions to us. Do your choices erode at what you had intended to become? Do they facilitate life? Do they reflect justice? Do they demean or elevate? Do they take or give? Are they self-indulgent or self-giving? Are they commensurate with your promises and life commitments, or do they confuse and tear apart relationships and people?

Something in all of us wants a theology that gets us "off

the hook." We don't want to face the reality that with freedom comes responsibility, that our actions impact not only ourselves but also those around us either for good or for ill. Examine the results of your own and others' choices. Is there nurture, joy, peace, growth, selflessness, health, well-being, reconciliation, maturity, mutuality or healing? Or is there discomfort, resentment, disillusionment, disharmony, incompleteness, greed, emptiness, bitterness, calloused emotions, selfishness, impatience or hurt?

Paul reminds us of our call to life-giving behaviors in his admonition to the Christians at Philippi. "Finally, brothers, whatever is true, whatever is noble, whatever is right, whatever is pure, whatever is lovely, whatever is admirable—if anything is excellent or praiseworthy—think about such things" (Philippians 4:8).

There is still much to be said—and discussed—about the issues of life-giving behavior such as motivation (Why do I want to be life-giving in the first place? How are life-giving choices made in the light of our addictive natures?); control (What if someone is getting away with something I'm sure is wrong?); and teaching (Can you encourage pure behavior without eliminating ambiguity?). A biblical theology of sexuality and ethics begins with a relationship, not arbitrary moral dictums, with a Creator who is passionately in love with his creations, with a Creator who longingly seeks and urges their well-being. This theology comes full circle and ends in a relationship with that same God embracing his creatures and thereby encouraging them to choose to live a life of well-being and wholeness.

This is not a cosmic quiz show where an angelic audience waits anxiously for the earthling contestant to beat the clock, where the odds to answer the game-winning questions permit the person both to save his or her reputation with a national TV audience (What will they think?) and to drive away in a brand-new Buick. The person who knows the answers wins the prize—or so we were told.

God is not the dispassioned director, sitting in the production booth hoping for an entertaining performance with an obligatory remark that "may the best man win." This life-giving theology is full of passion, individual concern,

struggle, ownership, responsibility, forgiveness and confrontation. Our attempts at closure, distancing and
removing the ambiguity strip the gospel of its relational
core and betray our secret desire for control—a control that
would lift us above the fragile nature of real human choices. This theology is about a God who's crazy enough to
want to be our friend, a God who doesn't quit, a God who
is faithful and a God who knows that rules break but people tear.

► *Discussion Questions*

1. How does your view of God influence the way you
view his commandments (pages 101-102)?

2. What is meant when we say God's commandments fit
life's design (pages 100-106)? Explain how "Thou shalt" can
be translated to "Everyone ought." Give an example of a
commandment that illustrates this idea.

3. How do we make promises with our bodies by the
choices we make (pages 105-106)? Are such promises inherent
in what it means to be human? Why or why not?

4. What are life-giving behaviors (pages 106-108)? List
synonyms to describe or define life-giving behaviors. How do
these descriptions or definitions alter or support your relationship with God?

►SECTION THREE:

Personal Filters

Introduction

" 'Not at my table, Martin Gregory! Wipe that
grim look off your face and enjoy your lunch!'
"I did enjoy it. I enjoyed the easy talk we
made, the cautious affection we exchanged. Of
course it was a pretending game: Let's pretend
there isn't any time but now, that we can be just
good friends, that I don't have a wife and two
children and that, here in this room, I can hardly
remember their faces. I remembered something
else, however. An old uncle who was very kind to
me made one day a strange kind of confession:
'Martin, I've been lucky. I've never met a woman
I wanted more than my wife. I've often wondered what would have happened if I had.'
Something of what I was thinking must have
shown in my face, because quite abruptly, Laura
asked the question:
" 'What really brought you here, Martin?' "[1]

So much for biblical theory; now what do we do? Theory will not be all that helpful to me as a single man on her
couch in the middle of a passionate embrace, or after a romantic interlude during which we overlook the bluffs of

Laguna Beach and share a bottle of our favorite wine. Theory will not help me as a married man sitting in a counseling session with a beautiful woman who hints of her availability, or when the sexual relationship within my own marriage grows predictable and boring, prompting a more attentive awareness of greener pastures and a sometimes volatile fantasy life. Nor does theory seem helpful when I struggle with my impotence, my wife's frigidity or our inability to communicate our sexual needs, wants and fears. Theory doesn't help when as a divorced single person I am faced with the realities of a dating world that assumes sexual intercourse is the dessert portion of a first date's four-course meal. Nor does the theory seem to remove the dilemma created by my ambivalence regarding my sexual orientation.

Theory doesn't seem particularly helpful in the other areas of my ethical indecision such as when I'm given the choice between staying at the office or spending time with my family; facing the need to lie to cover my tail; feeling envious as I look at my neighbor's new Porsche; or wondering whether working for a company that practices unethical business dealings makes me a co-conspirator if I choose to remain silent. I know what I believe. But . . . the questions become clear: How do I translate theory into practice? How can my belief system move into the world of everyday moral choice-making? What about those gray areas of life?

We all have "decision-making filters"—grids through which our decision-making processes pass. We say things such as "The devil made me do it." "Who cares?" "The Bible told me so." "What would my mother say?" "It wasn't intentional." "If it's okay for the president of the United States, then it's okay for me." "But we love each other." "If I do, I'll burn in hell."

Our filters are our reasons for doing what we do. They connect who we are to our decision-making. A look at our filters begins to reveal our motivation—the belief system, the heart—that is the foundation to our moral choices.

Decision-making filters also reveal what we do with the issue of responsibility—our continual struggle with being a

victim or a fighter in the area of moral choices. Understanding our decision-making filters is necessary because a faulty
filter skews the way we understand biblical foundation. Jesus was always careful to create the right context for his
comments. He knew that when his hearers listened through
an inadequate filter, the questions they asked weren't always the real questions they wanted answered. And, in
truth, our ethics will only be as good as our decision-
making. In other words, does the *what* match the *why*?

In the first section of this book we focused on who
owns us and how that determines our moral choices. We
also talked about how our choices are linked to our identity. In Section Two, we linked our beliefs about our identity
to our beliefs about God and sin and the world. Is reality
capricious and arbitrary, or gracious and benign? In Section Three, we will continue to link our sexuality with our
identity. We will ask ourselves: In what way does our identity create a decision-making filter? How does that filter
translate our theory—or theology—into practice? Where does
responsibility fit into the area of moral choice-making?
Why do we do what we do?

CHAPTER 7

Making Choices: No Longer Victims

"All behavior stems from decisions we make, not simply from our urges and drives and feelings."—Keith Clark[1]

■ ■ ■

Father: But he's a married man.
Daughter: I know, Pop. We're just working together, that's all.
Father: I'm worried about you.
Daughter: It just happened, Pop.
Father: That's how we make decisions. We just let them happen.
—Paraphrased from the movie *Violets Are Blue*

Every time I remember that poignant scene between the concerned father and his confused daughter, I experience the impact of the father's final words. This same scene is repeated over and over again in movies, on soap operas and in real life as individuals allow life just to happen. Assuming they are victims to what life has to offer, people offer no resistance to what's happening in their lives and the lives of those around them.

But choices are the stuff of real life. The primary task of our life is making choices. But choices are made all the more difficult in a world where options seem limitless. As Madison Avenue seductively presents its different options, we believe we're promised the good life. We also hope Michelob is right and we can in fact "have it all."

Our choices are made even more difficult by our desire to be in control. We make every attempt to rise above the vulnerability that comes with responsibility. We try to eliminate ambiguity, the process of reducing life to black and white. And we continue to hone our art of moralizing in hopes that we will look better if someone else looks worse.

As part of the postponed generation, we're good at avoiding choices. Life is a wait-and-see proposition, and we live much of it by default, substituting immediate gratification for priorities or long-term commitments. As young adults, we live in a world where we're enticed by a rapidly developing preoccupation with the American dream, with its lifestyle of opportunity and ease. Its clear, but often subconscious, message is that we do indeed have a right to happiness and personal worlds relatively free from discomfort and sacrifice. Unless, of course, we choose to sacrifice our family and friendships for the sake of business and monetary success.

Our obvious tendency toward postponement and preoccupation with self is being challenged and fueled by the world around us. With the continued threat of a nuclear holocaust and the emerging possibility of self-genocide through an AIDS epidemic, we need to understand that life invites us to make difficult decisions that affect the health of people and relationships for this and future generations.

At the same time, we feel continually pulled toward self-preservation. This is a more sophisticated selfishness than the self-actualization of the late '60s and early '70s, which lived off the theme "Let's live for today." The self-preservation of the late '80s is more cautious and displays its selfish nature by trying to acquire perfection in our possessions, as an attempt to avoid the mess in our emotional lives.

But our consumer society has lied to us; it's offered us goals that are, at best, cruel and deceptive. We have assumed that life can be understood, controlled and even conquered. An insightful Indian noted, "Americans have a tendency to view everything in life as a test; win and lose are the only options we know." The result is a fear of boredom, sadness and ordinariness—anything that indicates the possibility that we may have failed. It's no wonder our culture fears impotence, for we see it as a charge against our ability to be powerful and in control. Our preoccupation with achievement has left us empty, hoping that the next fad, how-to book, lecture series, or perhaps a prince or princess will come to the rescue.

We are a culture driven by unreal expectations and consequent addictions. As a result, we walk through life with an unstable identity structure, succumbing to anything that promises relief from the dread of being ordinary. Always needing more, we continually focus on what life isn't, on what we don't have and on what we know we need. Life is divorced from today and consequently from any choices or commitments we have made in favor of that perfect option that is just around the corner.

Our understanding of sexuality and the moral choices we make must be examined against the backdrop of this cultural pressure. Our need for perfection, closure and immediate happiness has only served to enforce a system in which we have become victims in the area of ethics. On one extreme, we amputate our sexual urges and drives, believing our ability to control such desires will alleviate any need to struggle with difficult decisions. And at the other extreme, we assure ourselves we have a right to personal pleasure in a world where consenting adults is the only rule.

► *Making Choices and the Temptation to Be a Victim*

Let's examine these two extremes more closely. The first extreme is an illusion of control. When we choose by first eliminating some options, our illusion has its price. We fail to understand the power of repression and the way repressed needs and desires are acted out in unhealthy ways. So afraid are we of our irrational side that we deny its existence. When options are repressed, desires eventually surface and we express surprise. "That's not like me. I don't know where that came from," we report, as if some alien power has temporarily taken custody of our body.

The second extreme is the illusion that life just happens. No less costly, this illusion is also set against a backdrop of our assumed right to happiness and argues from feigned naiveté. "I didn't consciously seek to hurt anyone" is the way one young woman phrased her feelings after a negative encounter.

A decision made by determining one's needs and desires can easily evolve into a position of dependence— needing someone else to meet those needs and consequently make one happy. Songs in the Top 40 invite us to "feel all right." But only when we're "with the one we love tonight." The result? People are "inclined to abdicate to someone else the responsibility for their own happiness, particularly their happiness in relationships. A lot of us wait for other people to behave in ways which will make our relationships with them fulfilling. And that's a mistake."[2]

Life doesn't just happen, nor can it be neatly confined. Whether we like it or not, our identity is made up of the commitments we have made. If we are responsible and believe we have the right to choose, we can make commitments, covenants or pledges. Such commitments assume we are not victims of life nor are we victims of our irrational, dark and evil side. In the words of Eugene Kennedy: "We have our own responsibility for an interesting life. We literally have to give a damn and not just allow life to happen to us."[3]

There is a two-step process at work here. First, we need to face that expansive reservoir of sexual drives and needs that makes up our identity. We need to stop again to remind ourselves that sex, or sexuality, isn't just intercourse. Sex is more than what happens with our genitals; it is the full range of what it means to be male or female with all our emotions, needs and drives. This definition is important—and worth repeating—because it implies that the issue of sexual ethics is not resolved by what we do, or don't do, about intercourse.

By facing our own sexual drives and needs, we take responsibility for our own choices and what it means to be a body-person. In addition, we give ourselves permission to get to know that part of our identity—namely our needs, insecurities, drives and urges—that has remained, for the most part, hidden or repressed. If accepting our sexuality means embracing the full range of our humanness, then we are compelled to get to know our hidden self—the irrational needs, the impulses and the obsessions. We begin to question. Is it possible that our emotions, feelings, drives and urges are user-friendly? Can there be options other than repressing, ignoring, being victimized or acting out? If we are still loved by God regardless of what he sees in our hidden self, does that love give us permission to embrace our incompleteness and our imperfection? Would that kind of love make a difference in the way we make decisions?

The second step of this process is to accept the fact that we have permission to choose. We are given permission to own who we are with our full range of needs and desires. We are also given permission to choose behaviors that are healthy for ourselves and for those around us. We are created with a capability and a freedom to make choices, and we have the option to make healthy or unhealthy decisions. While we may argue over the health of our choices, we begin with this one non-negotiable fact: We must make choices. If we are to live a healthy, moral, human life, we must choose that kind of life. None of us is a victim. And there are two implications of this fact that apply to all of us:

1. We are not islands. Whether we like it or not, we are connected. And our choices link us relationally. That's the price we pay for living as humans. Our nature portrays our relational bent. Love, trust, respect (including self-respect), affirmation and nurture—all find meaning in the context of relationships. Our choices take on meaning because they have the power to build up or tear down. This means that in relationship with one another, we can literally make a difference. We don't just occupy space, mingle or cross paths. By our choices we assist one another toward becoming either gods and goddesses or creatures of horror.[4]

With our connectedness come responsibility and consequences. But how do we learn that lesson without an accompanying demand for perfection or a guilt-laden preoccupation with "What should I do?" Is this just another call to morality shaped by fear, a call to perfection while walking on eggshells? The issue of responsibility touches our understanding of freedom. Unfortunately, we assume that the call to moral responsibility eliminates our freedom. But, as we noted in Chapter 6, commandments do not eliminate freedom; neither does the call to responsibility. We find we are not only free "from," but we are free "to." Our freedom comes precisely when we recognize our boundaries and show respect for the bonds we've chosen as part of the relationships to which we're committed.

Wedding ceremonies symbolize this kind of choice— this exchange of freedom "from" for freedom "to." To my spouse, I promise "to be wholly yours, to cleave only to you, to provide an environment that nurtures you, where there is trust and you can blossom, where the giving of our bodies enhances the previous giving of ourselves." My commitment, choice or bond creates a boundary that offers me the freedom to make life-giving choices for myself and that special person (in this case, my spouse) with whom I am in relationship.

We have all made such commitments. They may be conscious or subconscious. They may be verbal or nonverbal. They may be public or private. But they are nonetheless commitments—decisions about the direction or path of our lives and our relationships. These commitments may be relative to celibacy, marriage, faithfulness, exclusivity in a relationship, a pledge of confidentiality or simply an affirmation of friendship.

Such commitments offer not only the freedom "from"

alternatives (which may in fact be good or healthy choices), but also the freedom "to" fulfill and protect. We must remember that the issue of choice is not simply to eliminate other options. To illustrate, Andrew Greeley reminds us that "restraining fantasy [or freedom "from"] does not mean eliminating it, and renouncing genitality . . . does not mean . . . that one ceases to have sexual hungers or that one is immune from appraising members of the opposite sex as potential genital partners."[5] It means that because of our commitments, we are free to choose behaviors that nurture and develop those commitments and relationships without denying that other options exist.

It doesn't take long before we realize if we're not choosing behaviors that nurture and protect our commitments, we can easily become victimized by unhealthy and unwise choices and behaviors. By not making choices that favor our previous commitments—namely intimacy, mutual nurture and wisdom—our underlying desires take control and we feel we're being victimized. ("I just couldn't say no" or "I had no intention of hurting anyone," we confess.) These behaviors become addictive while the underlying hunger for intimacy remains unfulfilled. Feeling guilty, confused or wishing for more discipline, we work harder to repress what is already there or pretend that it doesn't matter.

Another freedom afforded to one who embraces a commitment is the freedom to enter fully into life. There's a cultural temptation to believe that life happens only when we keep all our options open. But it seems all choices of life and love bring with them a predicament. On the one hand, we need to practice individuality and freedom. On the other hand, we need boundaries to protect our intimacy and vulnerability. "Americans are . . . torn between love as an expression of spontaneous inner freedom, a deeply personal, but necessarily . . . arbitrary choice, and . . . love as a firmly planted, permanent commitment, embodying obligations that transcend the immediate feelings or wishes of the partners in a love relationship."[6]

Only when we fully embrace the vulnerability of putting ourselves on the line, making a choice, standing by a commitment—fully embracing the loneliness or intimacy that comes with such a moment—do we embrace life. In those moments we find God concrete. This God lives in the trenches of ordinary life. God lives with real people filled with the full weight of their fear, neediness and a longing for intimacy. They have the freedom to make choices that create an environment of health. By such choices, "quite ordinary people retain enormous power to heal each other. They do this by perceiving each other as total persons. When they love each other fully as human beings they are helping each other in many aspects of their personalities without even directly trying."[7]

2. We cannot have it all. As relational creatures confined by our contingent freedom, sooner or later we come face to face with the reality that we can't have it all, nor can we pretend to be above it all. All of us are incomplete people in a broken world. Our navigating through this world is contingent upon our making choices.

But in a culture saturated with its demands for personal rights, we wonder if our sexual desires have a right to be fulfilled. Encouraged by television, magazine advertisements and billboards, we choose to make fulfillment of desires—or the right to happiness—our goal for life. We may have other questions. Do any and all of our "normal" desires have a right to be fulfilled? At what expense? Is that healthy? Is there a difference between happiness (desire fulfillment) and maturity (desire channeling)? C.S. Lewis assures us that "the sexual appetite, like our other appetites, grows by indulgence. Starving men may think much about food, but so do gluttons . . . Surrender to all our desires obviously leads to impotence, disease, jealousies, lies, concealment, and everything that is the reverse of health, good humor, and frankness. For any happiness, even in this world, quite a lot of restraint is . . . necessary."[8]

We may want to believe the Michelob promise that we can "have it all," but eventually someone loses. Germaine Greer, a former proponent and now a survivor of the sexual revolution, remarked in an interview: "I believe that the permissive society was not really liberated at all. Great lovers know how to restrain themselves. I find love poetry more erotic than pictures of genitals—so perhaps now I'm considered a silly old virgin."

At this point it's important to note the close connection to the addictive process. When our identity has been lured by a person, behavior or substance that promises okayness, happiness and security, it's like a carrot on a stick. The addiction provides us with a source of life while protecting and removing us from the very life it promises to provide. We feel stuck, unable to escape our predicament. We want release, but we believe we need the "fix" to be okay. Guilt only intensifies our craving for the addictive fix—the substance, activity or person that can save us or make us feel okay.

To continually reprimand or even encourage more discipline for a person who is locked into an addictive behavior pattern is pointless. When a person who repeats negative behavior patterns announces "I can handle my problem" and then finds a need to lie, the symptoms of addiction are evident. The solution lies in recognizing that no one substance, activity or person has the power to meet all our needs. We need to realize that our okayness is intact apart from our need to fulfill any or all of our desires. We need to understand that if we are loved, we are free to make healthy choices, not choices based on a fear of punishment or a hope for reward.

What's at stake is that our health is predicated on our choices. When I'm obsessed it seems I can't resist a sale of any kind (any choices are difficult to make). Our journey to health necessitates an understanding of our identity being intact in the hands of a faithful God and our permission to make choices on the basis of that truth.

But if health is making choices that nurture health, then how do we handle the fact that life by its nature brings with it necessary losses? "We grow by losing and leaving and letting go," writes Judith Viorst. "We give up in order to grow. For the road to human development is paved with renunciation. Throughout our life we grow by giving up."9

Every life offers more possibilities than people can explore. Individuals have to restrict themselves and constantly "give up something in order to get something else. There is an inescapable, permanent, and occasionally frustrating necessity to make selections. In short, our lives are made up of innumerable individual choices according to some basic set of priorities."[10]

Let's examine an illustration of a man named Paul. "My wife only goes through the motions," he says. "I know she doesn't feel anything toward me sexually, and I'm tempted to pursue a young lady at my office who I know likes me. What should I do?" When Peter Kreitler tells this story, he puts Paul's dilemma in the context of his choices:

1. He could accept the situation as it was. Cost: no sex at the level he desired. Promise: living with a good wife, mother and companion.

2. He could choose to have an affair. Cost: might jeopardize his marriage. Promise: better and more frequent sex.

3. He and his wife could get medical and emotional support. Cost: there might be the immediate pain of hearing things that are hard to hear. Promise: both partners would be working toward a mutually satisfying and acceptable sexual relationship.[11]

Losing and letting go—we live life under the reality that choices and commitments must be made, in fact have already been made, by each of us. We have questions "about value, about what is really worth having . . . what is really worth keeping and what is really worth living or dying for. We have decided whether it's more important to be free than to be comfortable, more important to keep our marriages together than to find fantastic love on the side, more important to be honest than to make a quick buck—and we have made a thousand other decisions about what is really good."[12]

Our frustration comes from our being divorced from an understanding of a gracious reality. If reality is not gracious, then there is no reason for abstaining; life is unfair, and it might as well be everyone for himself or herself. But again, there's a price to pay. Listen to Clark: "The only alternatives

I see to [losing or letting go or] accepting even death are to become cynical about life because its great moments don't last, or to set out on a pursuit of self-fulfillment by doing all it takes in order to attain all that I crave. Cynicism doesn't appeal to me; and I've yet to meet a person always in hot pursuit of self-fulfillment who shows any real signs of being happy."[13]

This isn't another lecture on self-discipline for the sake of self-discipline. We must remind ourselves that our discussion doesn't begin with us—our decisions about sexual behaviors or even our decision to be good—but with God. "One begins by talking about God's fidelity to us and then . . . suggesting that such fidelity gives us both the strength and the motivation we need for the admirable but extraordinarily difficult human quality of faithfulness."[14] Then we can make choices that reinforce commitments and health, even in the midst of our confusing world that bombards us with its invitation to let life just happen.

▶ Discussion Questions

1. "That's how we make decisions. We just let them happen" (page 115). Do you agree or disagree with this statement? Explain. Think of an illustration where this has been true for you.

2. How does our culture set us up to be victims in the area of choice-making (pages 116-117)? Have you struggled with feeling like a victim in what's going on around you? If so, explain how you've handled those struggles.

3. If we are not "islands," how do our choices and commitments link us relationally (pages 119-122)? Think of illustrations in your own life or experience in which you've chosen to be free "to." What kinds of feelings did you experience from this freedom to enter fully into life?

4. What does it mean when we say, "We cannot have it all" (pages 122-123)? How does the addictive process influence our choices? How does your addiction to a person, an activity or a substance affect your choices?

5. Making healthy choices necessitates some loss (page 123). Think about a choice you've made that involved loss. How did you feel when you made that choice? How do you feel now? List those ways in which you gained health by making such a decision.

CHAPTER 8

Legalism: Morality by Law

In a Peanuts cartoon, Charlie Brown is sitting in a chair reading. His sister Sally is sitting in front of him, on the ottoman, attempting to undo the knots in her shoelaces.

"Stupid knots! Shoelaces drive me crazy!" she erupts.

Without being asked, Charlie begins his big brother monologue. "Grampa told me something about shoelaces and World War II. He said all the enlisted men were issued two pairs of shoes, but a lot of the men wore only one pair so they could keep the other pair shined and looking nice under their bunks . . . Battalion headquarters decided that the men should alternate shoes each day, and to make sure they did, the men had to lace their shoes in a certain way . . . One day they had to wear the shoes that had the laces crossed, and the next day they had to wear the shoes that had the laces going straight across."

Sally, looking increasingly perplexed, asked, "How did they ever win the war?"

When we worship rules or when rules become more important than the issue, we encounter a decision-making filter, a grid through which we make decisions. We filter our theology and our belief system through the same grid we use to view reality and the world. We set up morality as if it were a paint-by-number project.

When we introduced this section of the book, we affirmed morality as personal, something that cannot be divorced from who we are as people, including our spiritual nature and the personal commitments we make. We discovered that our moral decisions do not just happen; our choices are not made in a vacuum. We are not victims. Choices, whether they are conscious or subconscious, can only be understood when we look honestly at the belief systems that form them. We'll begin examination of our decision-making filters with a look at legalism.

What do the rules say? That's where legalism's decision-making filters begin. In a Christianized form, the question, "What does the Bible say?" is translated to mean, "What do the didactic, or the imperative, portions of the Bible say?" For if we can define the rules clearly and precisely, we can understand morality. What begins as a need and appreciation for the structure of rules becomes an enslaving and damaging belief system about life itself. What begins as a framework for our freedom becomes itself a relentless tyrant. What went wrong?

We said earlier that life is not a play without a plot. The Creator of life, because of his passionate interest in the well-being of his creation, speaks with regard to our ethical lives. And when he speaks, his commandments fit life's design. Our nature portrays us as having a bent toward a need to be healthy. Every game, even the game of life, has rules. "Rules belong to life the way the scale belongs to music. And the way grammar belongs to writing. We cannot live the moral life without rules any more than we can make music without scales. Or write a story without grammar."[1]

Rules, then, are not the issue. For some rules, as we have said, are a natural part of creation. In a helpful little book titled *Choices,* Lewis Smedes sheds some light on the positive nature of moral rules. He defines a moral rule as a "statement that tells us what we ought to do." But he also says: "Rules are not sacred or even good in themselves. They are means, not ends. We are obligated by the rules because we ought to live the kind of life that ends in happiness for others and ourselves."[2] This shift of seeing rules for the sake of rules and rules as a means to an end is part of the developmental process in all of us.

In Jean Piaget's discussion of moral development in *The Moral Judgment of the Child,* he talks about the move toward maturity that happens when we understand that being good no longer means simply obeying the rules. Maturity—or internalization—"comes to mean sharing in the responsibility of evaluating and making rules which will be fair to all, so that we can all enjoy living in a fair and just society."[3]

The trouble begins when we come to rules with our own emotional baggage and unstable identity structures. Legalism tries to avoid facing that unstable identity; it attempts to control life—to rise above the struggle, to make it black and white, nice and neat. Legalism tries to confine morality to strict behavioral issues. Rules become our justification. Legalism is above ambiguity where morality is obvious and unmistakable, where rhetoric is self-righteous and easily dispensed. Legalism is rationally manageable and becomes our ticket or guarantee of purity. Our identity is exonerated by rules, for the rules are no longer commandments that fit and encourage life. Legalism sees rules as ends in themselves.

Let's look at four characteristics of legalism—this decision-making filter that constricts rather than encourages health.

1. Legalism defines life by righteous limitations.
Legalism projects a line that divides right from wrong. Stay on the right side of the line, and you are affirmed for your virtue. Stray to the wrong side of the line, and you may jeopardize your good standing with God. This system encourages techniques for manipulating divine approval. It is

self-worth via comparison—retaining some corner in our lives where we're unscathed by the "scarlet letters" that identify the majority who seem incapable of rising above their temptations.

The Legalistic View

The line that divides

Right	from	**Wrong**
That which is good or allowed: • Earns divine approval. • Follows all rules to the letter.		That which is bad or not allowed: • Cannot attain divine approval. • Doesn't follow the rules.

The concern of legalists is right and wrong. They (Or should I say we?) are seeking to be exonerated by the rules. The issue is not what is right, but, "What can we get away with and still know that God loves us?" Or more realistically, "What can we get away with and know that we will still go to heaven?" As legalists, our identity is in a precarious position because our "okayness" is dependent upon our ability to stay on the right side of the line. The result? We become moral lawyers, living life as close to the line as possible while we continually move up and down looking for loopholes.

I can think of several illustrations of approaching life through the belief system of legalism. The first is from a book in which the author encourages his readers to avoid "premarital intimacy." (His language equates intimacy with genital sex.) In addition, the author devises a physical relationship scale of 1 to 10, in which 1 is "look" and 10 is "sexual intercourse." (To illustrate his thinking, 8 is "fondling breasts" and 9 is "fondling sexual organs.") When asked about the purpose for this scale, he responds that he simply presents this chart to the man first. He asks, "What is the maximum number you have been to as a couple?" Then he asks the woman if that is correct. If the relationship has gone beyond a number 7 ("French kiss"), the couple is asked to do additional homework by filling out a worksheet on moral purity. And, if they reach an 8 ("fondling breasts"), the man is expected to contact the instructor within 24 hours of the transgression. Repeated transgressions may terminate their training. It's not that I disagree with this author's intentions or his desire to prevent premature physical relations. I just don't believe ethics can be regulated by the good intentions of a leader or reduced to a neat system of restrictions.

Another illustration comes from a friend who retells this conversation from a premarital counseling session. "How are you doing in the area of sex?" he asked the couple.

"We're doing just great," was the reply. "In fact, we haven't had any problems."

Wanting to pursue such a bold statement, he inquired as to the reason for their success. "Oh, it's simple," said the young man. "We've divided our bodies into zones. She has four zones, I have three. I'm allowed to touch her one and two zones, but not her three and four zones. She's allowed to touch my one and two zones, but not my three zone."

Holding back his disbelief (and laughter), he asked, "And is that working?"

"Well," the young man paused, "we haven't crossed over any zone lines. But I guess there are times when we drive each other nuts."

When I heard this story, I couldn't help but think of my own attempts at "zoning." Like a lawyer, I too spent my energy going up and down the line, looking for that precious loophole.

Expanding our context for illustrations, the following story shows how legalism has even affected professional football. Because of the growing concern over the safety of quarterbacks, management devised a new rule to protect them. Previously, pass rushers could take two steps before making contact with the quarterback after he had thrown the ball. And in some cases they could legally slam him to the ground. Presently, the rule allows only one step. The irony is that most hits that occurred previously were legal. In other words, by the time the pass rushers had taken their second step, they had hit and sometimes injured the quarterback. Most of the time it appeared they could have pulled up, but they didn't. Why? Because they didn't have to; the hit was legal. So the rule was changed; it was made tighter and more restrictive. But that didn't work because players had discovered the loophole and could justify their destructive actions. By the rules, they had done nothing wrong.

Stories from my own history filter through my mind, reminding me how ingrained I am in the belief system of legalism. I remember being a part of my church's youth group in high school and learning morality on a scale of 1 to 10. The conversations my friends and I had about sexual behavior were predictable. "Is it okay to pet if she has a sweater on, but not okay if it's a T-shirt?" "Is it okay to French kiss as long as we come up for air every 60 seconds?" "Is it okay to give a body hug as long as there's a Bible between us?" "Is it okay to masturbate as long as you fantasize about someone ugly?" And the expected, "Is it okay to have intercourse with a woman if you're going to marry her?" Hoping the answer was yes, I tried to envision marriage with every woman I dated. Only in retrospect have I learned that the question wasn't even asked with legitimate concern for the woman, for me or for the issue of morality. It was asked as all legalistic questions are asked—for a means of protection. I was maintaining my righteousness before God at the expense of other people. Focused only on staying on the right side of the line, I used people in the name of purity.

In an insightful look at legalism and the issue of infidelity, Nancy Weber writes: "A kiss that lingers. A friendly pat on the fanny. When does lust become infidelity? . . . Have you been unfaithful lately? Maybe the answer, for all of us, lies somewhere between the spirit and the groin, between the doer and the done-to."

She goes on with tongue in cheek: "It wasn't a real infidelity if you wanted someone else (but it was if you asked for her telephone number). It wasn't a real infidelity to ask for her number (unless you called and arranged to meet on the sly). It wasn't a real infidelity to meet her on the sly (unless you kissed her). It wasn't a real infidelity to kiss her (unless she had the flu and you gave it to your wife). It wasn't a real infidelity to have a night full of luscious dreams starring naughty schoolgirls (unless you woke up

unhappy to find yourself in the nuptial bed). It wasn't a
real infidelity to do it with the old flame your wife knows
and likes (but it was to do it with the ex-wife she can't
stand). It wasn't a real infidelity to have a go with someone
you met while traveling on business (as long as you en-
dorsed your wife's romp with the pediatrician that night) . . .
It wasn't a real infidelity unless you fell in love. It wasn't a
real infidelity unless you fell in love and left home. It wasn't
a real infidelity unless you fell in love and left home and
took the kids. And the money."[4]

Legalism assumes that problems of sexuality can be
solved in terms of whom we sleep with and exactly how
we relate to each other physically; in other words, "How
far did you go on the physical relationship scale?"

Jesus encountered this ethical system regularly, and he
hated it. Why? Because it strips people of their dignity.
They become objects, or tickets, for our moral protection.
When our identities stay detached from life, perched pre-
cariously on the mountains of which we're self-proclaimed
kings, we anxiously look for ways to preserve our respecta-
bility via comparison.

**2. Legalism seeks salvation and self-worth in per-
formance and divine approval.** Our identity is tied to
our ability to perform, whether it's our ability to behave,
be good, achieve, accomplish or comply. Legalism, or
keeping our noses clean by following all the rules, encourages measuring individual worth by taking a look at one's
possessions. Looking good is of primary importance. Our
identities are at stake here. What will people think? What
will God think? Our thoughts hear the lyrics, "You better
watch out . . . You better not pout . . ."

A legalistic belief system is pervasive and addictive. It's
built on the faulty assumption that says our identity is at
stake unless we can prove our merit by mastering the
dance steps of correct behavior. The issue is impression
management—maintaining the right image, covering our
tail, using our ability to manage public opinion to remove
ourselves from any personal responsibility. It has led to
what one author called the "no-fault confession." Any

wrongdoing is deflected by arguing that the system was rigged, or by blaming someone else who stands between me and the sin committed, or by diverting the attention to the side of the scales that contains all the good and important things I've been doing for humanity. Consequently, confession becomes a time for performance reckoning. Our prayers begin with the words of the Pharisee: "God, I thank you that I am not like other men—robbers, evildoers, adulterers—or even like this tax collector" (Luke 18:11).

Legalism is a belief system fueled by fear. For with our identity at stake, we are continually in fear of what we need to protect and, consequently, of what we have to lose—our precious reputation. It feels like the old childhood game of King of the Mountain. All of our energy is diverted to protection, positioning and deflection. We have everything to lose and nothing to gain.

We have a list for what is wrong—that which produces death—so our logic tells us that if we avoid the items on this list we will live and be righteous. The Pharisees regularly asked Jesus to affirm their efforts at purity by recognizing what they didn't do. They hoped he would affirm the toil of their ever-active "inner bookkeeper" or at least give his name to their board of reference for their company letterhead. "Give me some reassurance about my herculean efforts to be good," the Pharisee in each of us cries. Like the Pharisees, we aren't prepared for Jesus' clear reply: "The list can't save you. You're already lost. Keeping score is not what's at stake here."

This struggle is not new, as illustrated by this widely circulated parable of the snake. "In the beginning God didn't make just one or two people; he made a whole bunch of us. He wanted us to have a lot of fun and said you can't really have fun unless there is a whole gang of you. So he put us all in this sort of playground park called Eden and told us to enjoy.

"At first we had fun just like he expected. We played all of the time. We rolled down the hills, waded in the streams, climbed the trees, swung on the vines, ran in the meadows, frolicked in the woods, hid in the forest and acted silly. We laughed a lot.

"Then one day this snake told us that we weren't having real fun because we weren't keeping score. When he explained it, we still couldn't see the fun. But he said that we should give an apple to the person who was the best at playing and we'd never know who was best unless we kept score. We could all see the fun of that for we were all sure we were the best.

"It was different after that. We yelled a lot. We made up new scoring rules for most of the games we played. We stopped playing other games such as frolicking because they were too hard to score.

"By the time God found out about our new fun, we were spending about 45 minutes a day playing and the rest of the time calculating the score. God was angry about that, very, very angry. He said we couldn't use his garden any more because we weren't having any fun. We said we were having lots of fun and we were. He shouldn't have got upset just because it wasn't exactly the kind of fun he had in mind.

"He wouldn't listen. He kicked us out and said we couldn't come back until we stopped keeping score. To rub it in, (to get our attention he said), he told us we were going to die anyway and our scores wouldn't mean anything. But he was wrong. My cumulative score is now 16,548, and that means a lot to me. If I can raise it to 20,000 before I die, I'll know I've accomplished something. Even if I can't, my life has a great deal of meaning because I've taught my children to score high, and they'll be able to reach 20,000 or even 30,000, I know.

"Really it was the life in Eden that didn't mean anything. Fun is great in its place, but without scoring there's no reason for it. God has a superficial view of life, and I'm glad my children are being raised away from his influence. We were lucky to get out. We are very grateful to the snake."

Robert Capon insightfully describes this self-made predicament. "If we are ever to enter fully into the glorious liberty of the sons of God, we're going to have to spend more time thinking about freedom than we do. The church, by and large, has had a poor record of encouraging freedom. She has spent so much time inculcating in us the fear of making mistakes that she has made us like ill-taught piano students: we play our songs, but we never really hear them because our main concern is not to make music but to avoid some flub that will get us in dutch. She has made us care more about how we look than about who we are."[5]

It is worth noting here that a corollary dynamic is also in effect. Because their (Or should I say our?) identities are dependent upon being approved by performance, many legalists perpetuate negative, hidden or closet lifestyles and then constantly live with guilt while repeatedly asking for God's forgiveness. Why? Because they have no other reference for God other than someone to whom they say, "I'm sorry." For the legalist, bad love is better than no love at all.

3. Legalism must always find the culprit. I've had many people complain to me about couples who were sleeping together. Why? Because these people wanted recognition for their own moral purity. If their concern was legitimate, they would have gone directly to the couple in question. Such a perspective leads to separatism, the ultimate in an us-versus-them view of reality. The world is a hostile place, we contend, and those who are not like us are of this world. "Circle the wagons! We must protect the innocent—those that are just like us."

To protect our moral purity, we must find others on which to deflect our guilt, anger and acrimony. It's the older-brother syndrome from the parable of the prodigal son. "I've busted my tail keeping my nose clean," we argue. "But look at him or her." Others are getting away with the very things for which we've secretly wished, and what's worse is they don't seem to be paying a penalty. Our focus on the enemy—the "other," the heathen, the backslider—keeps us from squarely confronting our own irrational and dark side.

4. Ministers, teachers and leaders become moral policemen. Christians who become expert lawyers by

finding the necessary loopholes are often awarded a leadership position for distributing the daily regimen of behaviors
and handing out awards of merit at the annual "Righteous
Brothers and Sisters Banquet." As moral policemen, we believe we are responsible for others' ("our people," we call
them) behaviors, and we take their failures personally. I know
how this feels because I have been a moral policeman, and
my desire for the moral purity of the group had more to do
with my own reputation than the well-being of the people
involved. Somehow, the moral shortcomings of any individual
in my group (or my church) was a reflection on me, and
again, on my inability to perform. It was an illusion of
control.

By assuming the role of moral policemen, we avoid
struggle and suffering. Because we fear ambiguity and
doubt, we feel we have to have an answer to every question. By eliminating ambiguity, we remove moral choices
from their relational context. Rightness is valued above
wholeness. We see "being right" as the positive end of the
continuum and anarchy (or no answers) as the negative extreme. In avoiding a balance between these two extremes,
we miss the tension that requires community involvement
and personal responsibility.

There is something comforting about legalism. It seems
to remove us from the messiness of true responsibility, acknowledgment of failure and confession—in fact, from our
humanness. We're able to engage in (and even enjoy) those
sins we find repulsive while we maintain our secure perspective of moralizing—or sermonizing—about those who
are unable to withstand temptation.

In such a light, we wonder why legalism is so pervasive. Capon helps us understand by his observation that
"religion always sells. You can get people to buy almost
any version of salvation-by-towing-the-line you want to
dream up . . . Because the world *wants* to feel guilty, and
the rulers of the darkness of this world are always happy to
bake up fresh batches of guilt to keep the troops in line."[6]

The situation is all too clear. Legalism cripples us. Our
hearts are constricted. Our approach to life is myopic. Focusing on the notes we might miss, we fail to learn how to

hear, feel or enjoy the music. We are taught what not to do with certain parts of our body, but we aren't taught how to treat another person with dignity. We aren't taught the values of tenderness, gentleness or compassion; therefore fear cripples us. Fear prevents us from really loving another.

But doesn't the Bible say we are to fear God? Yes, but to fear God doesn't mean we should be afraid of God. When we talk about the fear of God, we are not referring to fear as we use the word today, but to awe and reverence. Awe is similar to fear, but different in some ways. Awe inspires a feeling of being overwhelmed, of confronting someone or something much more powerful than ourselves. But awe is a positive feeling, an expansive feeling. Where fear makes us want to run away, awe makes us want to draw closer, even though we hesitate to get too close. Instead of resenting our own smallness or weakness, we stand open-mouthed in appreciation of something greater than ourselves.

I suppose it's easier to be a legalist. It's not easy to be told you're responsible for who you are and what you do. For this reason, "authentic religion should not listen to us when we say, 'This is too hard. Tell me what to do so that I don't have to figure it out for myself.' It should urge us to grow, to leave childish patterns behind even if we would rather remain spiritual children."[7]

Our view of God has been tainted, and it affects the way we make choices. Some of us see God as an unflappable bookkeeper, recording our every move and responding accordingly. We walk around with a permanent flinch, expecting God's slap to balance the scales for some indiscretion of the past. We even rationalize the negative things that happen to us as God's way of keeping us in line. Others view God as the great Big Brother in the sky who keeps that ever watchful eye for any mishap, slip-up or wrongdoing. Maybe it's comforting to see God as a nagging parent or a report card that keeps track of our achievements and failures and grades us for our performance. There's an element of control, as if we still have the capacity to impress God (and those around us) with how significant and good we really are. And if we find ourselves not all that impressive, we can always point to those around us who haven't scored nearly as high.

Without realizing it, we become increasingly more self-conscious and less relational. Again, we spend 45 minutes a day having fun—embracing life, loving friends, creating environments of nurture—and the rest of the day working out the score.

We find it unsettling to see God as "the divine power urging [us] to grow, to reach, to dare." This God says to "go forth into an uncharted world where you have never been before, struggle to find your path, but no matter what happens, know that I will be with you." For "like a father who is genuinely proud when his children achieve success entirely on their own, God is mature enough to derive pleasure from our growing up, not from our dependence on Him."[8] Kushner's description of God confuses the legalist in us. We continue to search for the applause we receive from playing all the right notes.

▶ Discussion Questions

1. "Some rules are a natural part of creation" (page 128). Explain this statement and list rules that might fall into this category.

2. Can you relate to the legalistic view illustrated by the line that divides right from wrong (pages 129-133)? Share a story or example that illustrates this "line" mentality.

3. Many of us are obsessed with a legalistic system that values performance, and then we spend most of the time justifying ourselves by what we haven't done (pages 133-134). Why are we drawn to a moral system that requires us to keep score?

4. In the legalistic system, what is the value of looking for a culprit (page 136)? How does this search affect your relationship with others? your relationship with God?

5. Have you ever been a moral policeman (pages 136-137)? Explain. Have you ever wanted someone else to be a moral policeman for you? If so, what were the dynamics of this situation? Is the moral policeman still a part of your relationship with God? Explain.

CHAPTER 9

Narcissism: Grab for the Gusto

"I would say, 'I know this is wrong and whatever,' and he would say, 'If you love him—and it is obvious that he loves you—isn't that what counts?' "—From *The New Other Woman* by Laurel Richardson[1]

An author once described a city famous for its entertainment as a place where everyone rushed at a frantic pace, as if they were all doing last-minute Christmas shopping except that none of them believed in Christmas. This is an apt description of our cultural viewpoint of romance and sexuality. Individuals in our society look for love like we look for bargains in a shopping mall. What we need is sacrificed for what we want. What is long-term is sacrificed for what is immediate. What is wise is sacrificed for what is gratifying. What is necessary is sacrificed for what is urgent. And what we have now is sacrificed for what we think we should have. Consequently, the world of love and romance is inhabited by people who come for reasons other than love and romance. Consequently, like ski slopes, the world of love and romance is crowded with people who come for reasons other than devotion to the sport.

Although legalism stands at one end of the decision-making filter and narcissism at the other end, the delineation is not always clear. Both extremes wage a continuous battle, all too often in our subconscious. Our self-righteousness gives way to a devil-may-care defiance of any obligation, only to be plagued by insistent guilt, and the cycle repeats itself. We are at war with ourselves.

There are no casual words in a discussion of morality; therefore, it's important to clarify our usage of the word "narcissism." There is a healthy narcissism that refers to a "person who is genuinely alive, with free access to the true self and his (or her) authentic feelings." In contrast, however, an unhealthy narcissism expresses itself in an individual who is enamored with an "idealized, conforming, false self," with the true self locked in "solitary confinement."[2] It is this unhealthy extreme to which we refer as the decision-making filter of narcissism.

Narcissism is a filter that's bartered daily on network television, highway billboards and the glossy ads in national magazines. Each advertisement seeks to amend our personal bill of rights to include the fairness of life, the rewards of consumerism and the happiness of the individual. As an expression of our pursuit of absolute personal freedom, the roots of narcissism reach deep, finding a home in the addictive nature of our culture and entwining themselves in our culture's glorification of the self. Even though we hesitate to identify ourselves as "narcissists," the fact remains that as a decision-making filter, narcissism shapes the way we think, the way we live and the way we make choices.

While legalism invites us to morally evaluate our lives in hopes that such an evaluation will generate well-deserved merit points or at least a favorable public opinion, cultural and personal narcissism finds that any moral evaluation would conflict with the sacredness of individual expression. This conflict creates a dilemma in our initiating any form of ethical introspection. Moral regeneration, no matter how it is labeled, will always be at odds with America's characteristic of pragmatism or self-indulgence.

We tend to approach the subject of narcissism from a legalistic framework, with moralism and finger pointing. As enlightened as we want to think we are, the temptation is real, and the need for such projection comes from our own fear of the unhealthy narcissism within us and fear of our own love affair with self-indulgence. We still have enough legalistic tendencies to believe that our confessions and fear will only bring divine reprisal; therefore, we opt to identify the culprit as what (or whoever) causes us to be narcissistic.

I hope we can avoid that kind of finger pointing here. For in truth, we are all susceptible to the promises and lure of self-indulgence. We all short-circuit our growth by opting either for further repression or sermonizing. Let's look at three characteristics of narcissism, the decision-making filter that stunts our humanness—or as Harold Kushner describes it, the choice "that causes us to work hard but condemns us to end up somewhere other than where we wanted to be."[3]

1. Narcissism assumes isolation. It was a simple remark, but loaded with implications. "It's just that someday I'd like to have my act together," she said to me, after recounting her continuing struggles with parents, male relationships and self-esteem. She added parenthetically, "Maybe then, I won't need anybody." Her emphasis was subtle but pervasive: The best of all worlds is self-sufficiency.

Narcissism is a philosophy of life, a mind-set, a belief system, a decision-making filter that makes self-sufficiency seem like the ultimate solution. It automatically (though perhaps not consciously) changes the question that precedes any of our moral choices. "The question 'Is this right or wrong?' becomes 'Is this going to work for me now?' Individuals must answer it in light of their own wants [and] . . . in terms of the costs it exacts and the satisfactions it yields."[4]

My assumed isolation confines my decision-making to whatever quenches my appetite and appeases me. One does not have to look far for illustrations. " 'The affair with

Carl was nice,' began a 27-year-old housewife, 'because I didn't have to be intimate. It was just good, clean, honest sex. Well, I don't know about its being honest, but it was fun.' "[5]

In isolation, sex—like other areas of moral choice-making—is assumed to be without emotional attachments. It's an automatic consequence of the assumption that my choices must be made in the vacuum of my self. In relationships, then, morality is decided on the basis of contractual exchange. Emphasis is placed on knowing your feelings and desires and being clear in communicating and negotiating. But there is a price tag. Unfortunately, commitments are at the mercy of individual needs. "In other words," says Kushner, "happiness is having no commitments, no one to answer to . . . no one whose needs or problems will ever get in your way or tie you down."[6]

To what do we appeal, then, to urge another to keep a commitment? Or are we at the mercy of whim? Enamored with our personal expression of freedom, we fail to see the implications. For if all of us have the right to be free of others' demands, it will be hard to form attachments. Any obligation will be seen as infringing on another's freedom. The implication of this attitude is that in sex, anything that feels good, as long as it doesn't harm someone else, is all right; nothing is forbidden and nothing is required.

How does the cycle continue? "I'll look out for my best interests, while the other person looks out for his." Where does this narcissism lead? Remember Cain's statement, "Am I my brother's keeper?" Kushner comments: "And what is Cain's punishment? He becomes a wanderer on the face of the Earth, with no place to call home, with no community to support or comfort him. The original looking-out-for-number-one man, like all of his descendants, is condemned to spend all of his days unconnected."[7]

2. Narcissism assures the right to happiness. Our culture assumes an inalienable right to happiness. As independent, self-sufficient entities, we have only our own experience, needs, urges and desires on which to form a framework for decision-making. Something is healthy, so our reasoning goes, if it is healthy for me.

Narcissism assumes we have absolute freedom. We are no longer confined by the contingencies of our woundedness, our vulnerability and our need to be connected through community. "If it serves love, it's okay" is the by-line of this philosophy of life. Whereas legalists like rules, narcissists say they prefer people. At first glance, this sounds good. The difficulty comes when we attempt to define love. If moral "oughtness"—the context of our sexuality—is called irrelevant or is at best defined by our own narcissism, where is the freedom in our choices toward others? Like legalists, aren't we still enslaved, though now by our own choices and subjectivism?

Absolute freedom assumes there are no limits or boundaries. "We went to bed because we loved each other," said one man who spoke in the same tone of voice as if he had just ordered an additional dessert because he loved chocolate. This narcissistic filter assumes it is our nature to be loving, kind and selfless. And that's where we're wrong. It is our nature to be selfish, to take care of our own needs first. And isolation only continues to encourage our selfishness—using people to maintain our hard-fought position as King of the Mountain. We must spend our lives learning what is unnatural—learning to need, receive and nurture without need of reward.

"You don't believe that premarital sex is just a blanket yes or no, do you? It's ultimately up to the individual, isn't it?" This narcissistic question was asked in a legalistic tone in pursuit of permission. Under the guise of personal freedom, the question admits enslavement to our need to be respectable and to appease our immediate urges. We've been tricked into believing that our passion knows best. We notice that in pursuit of that goal, we slowly sacrifice personal growth. We've failed to see that what we pursue is only projection.

We have clouded the issue further by culturally equating sex with happiness. Our self-sufficiency and right to happiness ironically have condemned us to a life of endless pursuit. One author notes: "Set up as a god, sexual pleasure calls the couple to an endless menu of sexual variations, yet often leaves them restless and bored despite their 'good sex life.' The sexual gourmet will experience many remarkable sensations, but will end up unsatisfied."[8] Immediate gratification is a natural consequence of our prison of self-sufficiency. We frantically look for the Christmas present that will satisfy, but we project a view of life that says Christmas is a myth.

Immediate gratification creates a dilemma in which it appears everything is at stake. "If we don't take advantage of this opportunity, our lives will never be the same." What we've missed is the bigger picture of life. All that matters is now, and all else is willingly sacrificed. Walter Trobisch illustrates the situation: "I want something. Not you, but something from you. *I don't have time to wait.* I want it immediately, without delay. It doesn't matter what happens afterwards . . . You are for me only the means by which I can reach my goal. I want to have it—have it without any further ado, have it, immediately."[9]

One author has said that when a man says he wants a "good woman," he is referring to an experience of sexual ecstasy. What he wants is a good sensation for which the woman is the necessary apparatus. Like the proverbial bluebird of happiness, we relentlessly pursue what we think we should want, only to find it all the more elusive. We fail to realize that when we begin to believe that any means justifies the end, we are losing control of our personal happiness.

Consequently, we celebrate our freedom by depersonalizing others. We look at them as objects that we can use for our own selfish purposes. The problem with this attitude is not that it corrupts, but that it desensitizes our emotions and distorts our perspective.

In order to maintain our illusion of happiness as a goal, we orchestrate our life to worship the ecstatic. Anything that titillates keeps us from facing our loneliness, our vulnerability and our need for connectedness. The mystery is removed. We worship ecstasy. The goal—or orgasm—is celebrated over and above the process. We equate lovemaking with intercourse and forget that it's the journey that matters.

3. Narcissism offers permission to be a victim.
While reading *The New Other Woman* (a candid look at the
dynamics surrounding the current phenomenon of contemporary single women in affairs with married men), I was
struck by the continued reference to the premise that a
woman doesn't consciously choose to become the "other
woman." In fact, most women explicitly deny any premeditation. While I realistically agree that most of us would
deny premeditation, we do ourselves a disservice when we
place responsibility for our moral choices on circumstance
or fate. "It just happened!" "I couldn't help myself." "I
never meant to hurt anyone." "I never intended to get involved." "I can't believe it really happened to me!" "It's
happening to everyone." When we make statements like
these, we are giving one another permission to be victims.
We're saying responsibility is optional. We're living with
the assumption that life simply happens, that our identity
boundaries are ultimately defined by our hormones and
desires.

The problem, according to advocates of this philosophy of life, is the removal of guilt. Guilt is what holds us
back from enjoying life and prevents our desires from
reaching full expression. I would certainly be the first to
agree that we have manufactured an overabundant stock-
pile of guilt through our cultural shoulds and oughts, but it
is a fallacy to argue that removal of this guilt will set us
free. For freedom is not the absence of boundaries. In the
words of a friend, "Eros is great. It just needs glasses."
Freedom is permission to be fully alive in a context that invites us to health, which means the freedom to say no as
well as yes.

Suzanne Britt Jordan explains: "No is a good word . . .
[It's] part of life. I think that doing without is not half as
bad as endless having. I think we could give our children a
lesson in something besides instant gratification. I think we
could put life back into sex, material possessions, good
times and people by treating all of them as precious rather
than disposable. Say no. Wait awhile. Think it over. Build
up the anticipation. Savor the possibilities. Skip it for now.
Have it later. Abstinence makes the heart grow fonder."[10]

We're a vulnerable generation. Our fear of intimacy is betrayed when we avoid the responsibility that comes with real relationships. We become prisoners in a world of freedom, a generation with limitless choices and no guidelines along the way. What's at stake is not simply convincing the narcissistic person of the error of his or her ways. It's not just that we're making wrong or sinful choices. As we've said all along, the issue is more than just behavioral.

What's at stake is an inadequate view of my identity. I've never been given permission to live life with boundaries, to invest, to be responsible, to commit, to treat life as precious. Believing that my identity is still vulnerable, and that I am caretaker of my own soul, I—the well-trained consumer—grasp at any hope that promises relief. My unstable identity finds itself lulled into passive obedience lured by any experience that offers temporary shelter. Then, all alone, in the solitary confinement of my own freedom, I shake my fist at an unfair world for never delivering the goods of happiness.

▶ Discussion Questions

1. How does our culture encourage unhealthy narcissism—a state of idealizing a false self while the true self is hidden in solitary confinement (page 142)? Think about how media, society and personalities can influence this self-indulgence.

2. Is it true that our culture prefers self-sufficiency (pages 143-144)? Why or why not? How does this self-sufficiency manifest itself in our society? What are the results? How do you deal with your own drive toward self-sufficiency?

3. In what ways are we taught that happiness is our right (pages 144-146)? Think about your own life. What people or things have suggested to you that you have a right to happiness?

4. "Freedom is not the absence of boundaries. Freedom is permission to be alive in a context that invites us to health, which means the freedom to say no as well as yes" (page 147). Explain what this means to you and how it applies to your own life.

5. Reread the last two paragraphs of this chapter. You are a part of this vulnerable generation that avoids responsibility because of its fear of intimacy. You have been identified as a prisoner in a world of freedom, an individual with limitless choices and no guidelines. Does this identification fit for you? Why or why not? Write your own identification of your generation and its view of sexuality.

CHAPTER 10

Life-Giving Choices

"We call people good because they add to the goodness of other people's lives. Morality is always about keeping life good, or making it better, or preventing it from getting worse than it already is. This is why it is good to be a good person. Not so that you get God to applaud you. But so that you do some good for your friends and neighbors, even for your enemies."—Lewis Smedes[1]

Life doesn't fit. At least not in the categories we use to contain, define and reduce it to manageability. Our choices are the same way; they don't always fit into life's categories. Life is about personal investment. We cannot be rescued by a series of moral analysis charts that gives us percentages on right or wrong choices. Something in us wants protection from the loss, energy and pain that come with our investment. We can do that with a carefully maintained book of rules that outlines a course of action for every life situation, or we can abdicate responsibility for whatever feels good at the time and let life happen. No matter which choice we make, personal investment is difficult.

That's what morality is about. It's about people, relationships and the commitments we make. Whether we like it or not, our identity is made up of the commitments we have chosen to make. When we make commitments, covenants or pledges, we assure ourselves we are not victims of life.

Morality is not a spectator sport. Either we have choices and can make commitments or we are at the mercy of our feelings, hormones, urges and drives that we act out or repress. We can approach life either as gallant fighters or as victims. Taken at face value, this perspective of morality can be an oppressive, unwanted burden. It seems to view life as a relentless contest in which we, the unsuspecting contestants, are victims of some cosmic joke. Those of us who are legalists take our role seriously (too seriously) and set out to prove we can win. We give up learning, risking, trying, failing, laughing and playing for keeping score. Something in us wants to win, and we set ourselves up for that task. Others of us who are narcissists see the contest as an opportunity to play out the scenario of the winner—"as the one who dies with the most toys."

Morality is personal; it's about who I am becoming as a person and who you are becoming as a person. Consequently, our choices are not arbitrary. They reflect me and you. Morality begins with who owns us, and it's who (or what) owns us that determines or creates our decision-making filter.

We've already looked at two decision-making filters: legalism and narcissism. And we're faced with the obvious dilemma: Now what? In looking at the alternatives, we agree with Smedes: "We cannot live by moral rules alone, not in a broken world, a crazy world where to obey one rule can compel you to break another and where being right according to the rules can be wrong according to what it does to people.

"We cannot live by results alone, either, not in a complex world where results that feel good today can go sour on us later, and where good results for some people bring disaster to others."[2]

Then what is our task? We must consider the facts and use our intelligence in light of the commandments to think about life and how we can best respond to others in wisdom and kindness without succumbing to the excesses of legalism or narcissism. Is it possible to be moral or good without being rigid? Is it possible to be human without being unprincipled? Is there more to ethics than a list of dos and don'ts? Can we assert our values without being authoritarian? And what about the vast areas of life and human behavior that have little to do with morality—the gray areas that cannot be confined by rules and reduced to chaos by unabated individualism? Is there another option?

We will describe this third decision-making filter as "life-giving." It is the ethical filter of Jesus, introduced to us in the Gospels. This filter says people are more important than winning, looking good, being right, feeling good or immediate gratification. The sanctity of human life is at stake. Jesus created a whole new context for ethical issues. He takes us to the heart of the good news: Ultimately, Christian faith is not in the ethics business at all, but in the identity business—the business of changing lives, making broken things new and mending fault lines that tear the soul. It is within this context—the good news that my identity has little to do with points earned or squandered—that I am given permission to make personal and relational investments. If I no longer need to protect the fortress built for my unstable identity, I can begin to give up my need to prove my worthiness by earning points for my morality. Maybe then I will no longer see the world as my playground, somehow exempt from connections with real people and real emotions.

Life-giving ethics is more concerned with tools for relationships than with answers. Its focus is on life—human, passionate, rich with contradiction and spice, heartfelt—and not on re-creating some script. From a recent interview in a popular contemporary magazine, a young woman confessed she had slept with only one man. When asked why, she responded, "Because I don't want to die." Was she responding to a fear of AIDS? Perhaps. A lingering fear of

God's ultimate wrath? Perhaps. Or had she made a conscious choice based on consequence and health? Viktor Frankl reminds us that "as long as a man [or woman] is . . . motivated either by the fear of punishment or by the hope of reward—or, for that matter, by the wish to appease the super-ego—conscience has not had its say as yet."[3] In other words, morality has not yet been internalized.

So what does this life-giving filter look like? What are its identifying characteristics?

1. The life-giving filter is a gift of grace. It's worth repeating that our theology begins with God's word about us, not our word about God. The same is true with our ethics. Even our attempts at morality and goodness are based on God's prior word about our worth. Life-giving ethics means living life "from" acceptance rather than "for" acceptance.

Grace calls the ill-taught piano student in each of us to hear the music of hope, investment, covenant, love, relationship and life. Grace lets us know that we can never leave the relationship with our Creator. After all, the essence of morality (or becoming whole) is relationship, not orthodoxy, or established law. For morality is not where you arrive, but the direction you are going; it is not a possession, but a journey. Some Christians believe the goal of our Christian life is sinless perfection. I couldn't disagree more. The goal of the Christian life is wholeness and completeness. What's the difference? Sinless perfection sees life as relentless, a victory to be won, an enemy to be subdued. We live this kind of life by continually glancing ahead at the payoff we will receive from our bookkeeper at our destination. It's little wonder that many of us who were raised with that kind of mentality have spent much of our lives neurotically concentrating on not sinning. We've missed the point.

Wholeness and completeness embrace life. We begin to see God incognito in the "day-liness" of life, in our ordinariness and our humanness, in the struggles, the choices and the failures. We see God in the process—the failure or success—of the choice itself, not as the unrelenting judge waiting to see our test results.

Yet the perfectionist in us continues to wonder, "Are we there yet?" Preoccupation with results or our destination robs us of celebrating the moment. Haven't we done the same thing with our moral choices and the Christian faith in general? We want to reach sanctification by noon! Our goal is perfection or bust! Our identity becomes dependent upon our arrival. Sure the Apostle Paul speaks about setting ourselves to the goal, but not as a measurement for our identity. The life-giving filter—grace—says that our identity is already intact.

Robert Capon helps us clarify our understanding of grace when he says: "The life of grace is not an effort on our part to achieve a goal we set ourselves. It is a continually renewed attempt simply to believe that someone else has done all the achieving that is needed, and to live in relationship with that person whether we achieve or not . . . The life of grace is . . . not even our life at all, but the life of that someone else rising like the tide in the ruins of our death. For us, it is simply Jesus . . . It is a love affair with an unlosable lover."[4]

Our identity, secure in the hands of a loving and faithful God, is set free to love and pursue life (regardless of our performance) and no longer needs to be a testing ground to verify our piety. Father Robert Drinan, a Roman Catholic priest who served as a representative to Congress, declined re-election when he received word that forbade priests from holding public office. Although some thought he merely responded to orders from his superiors, others saw his action in a different way. In the words of Harold Kushner: "He was saying that he knew who he was. Being a Jesuit priest was the core of his identity; everything else, however enjoyable or gratifying it was, was secondary . . . Had he tried to be a Jesuit sometimes and a Congressman sometimes, he would have lost the sense of integrity which comes with being the same person at all times and which was the secret of his strength."[5]

Too often we live as if the jury is still out on our identity. We expect the prosecution to uncover those secret behaviors that will ultimately sway the judge to render a verdict of condemnation. But, loudly and clearly, grace says: "You're now free. Free! Not when you arrive, but now. Therefore, you are safe knowing you're free to fail! And because of that freedom, you're also free to nurture others, to love and forgive, to feel sorrow and awe, to give and receive." We're no longer speaking of doing right; now we're talking about transformation. In the words of St. Augustine: "Before grace, we had no free choice about not sinning; the best we could do was want not to sin. But grace has the effect of making us not only want to do right, but also able to do it—not by our own powers, of course, but by the help of our Liberator."[6] We no longer have anything to prove with our behavior.

Jesus was clear that morality isn't an exercise in producing self-worth. No clause calls for our reform. Ironically, however, "even though grace makes no conditions about reform, it does—and not always conveniently—produce the conditions that induce reform. Grace works our restoration the way physical life works our healing, by producing a general tilt in the direction of health, by being a force for wholeness which, while it never forces, continually disposes us to become whole."[7] The focus changes because the issue is no longer on right and wrong. The issue (in the words of C.S. Lewis) is "like catching the infection of a person." Or more like playing a violin than studying musical theory.

But, we want to understand grace by reducing it to a couple of neat paragraphs. We want to compare grace to magic or medicine. We want to explain it away as some form of a payoff for services rendered or hard work delivered.

And we wonder, "What should we do now?" Maybe that's just it. Maybe we need to begin by doing nothing. Perhaps we need to stop and listen to the reality that we are safe. Not safe, *if* . . . not safe, *as long as* . . . not safe, *provided* . . . Add anything—even a single qualifier, even a single hedge—and you lose the gospel of salvation, which is just Jesus." Listen to this reality: "Christ died—without waiting for [any of us] to reduce [our] sins to the level of temptations."[8] Like recipients of a through-the-mail sweepstakes award, we read between the lines, looking for the disclaimer. But with grace, there is none. You can keep looking, but you won't find any.

The alternative to grace is the tyranny of self-consciousness that comes with either legalism or narcissism. With legalism, we are preoccupied with our ability to perform or our fear of failure. With narcissism, we are preoccupied with what we need to be happy. With both alternatives, we continually struggle to do enough or get enough to be okay. "The only lasting freedom from self-consciousness comes from a profound awareness that God loves me as I am and not as I should be, that he loves me beyond worthiness and unworthiness, beyond fidelity and infidelity; that He loves me . . . without caution, regret, boundary, limit or breaking point; that no matter what I do, He can't stop loving me."[9]

2. The life-giving filter gives us permission to love, not just get "off the hook." Because of grace, moral choices can be personal. We are not just free "from," but we are free "to." According to Keith Miller, "Jesus evidently didn't want people to neurotically concentrate on 'not sinning,' but rather to focus on loving God and people."[10]

Fidelity, then, can no longer be viewed as just "not sleeping around," but as nurturing and cherishing my spouse, my friend or the one to whom I am committed. This kind of behavior creates an environment of encouragement, so the other person will be better off for my having been with him or her. Chastity, then, can no longer be viewed as just "not going all the way," but as a lifestyle that models respect for others, a way of living that doesn't use people. It says, "I honor your dignity by the way I treat you." Honesty, then, can no longer be viewed as just "not lying," but as living truthfully, without using the truth to hurt others and without hiding behind a veneer of moral superiority.

A life-giving filter offers us the freedom to say yes to the sanctity of human life. "To be free in Christ means to be a person-with-Christ; and to be a person-with-Christ is to be a person-for-others."[11] We want others to be free; therefore, it's important to speak of freedom for others as well as for ourselves.

When we are free for others, we choose to love other human beings. We find fulfillment "in cherishing and nurturing others even when it costs us something, and whether or not we get something out of it. It is the respectful, non-possessive, non-manipulative, nurturing and accepting of the beloved which makes human fulfillment possible."[12]

The Bible has no sex ethic. It presents only a love ethic that may be consistently applied to the sexual mores dominant in any given country, culture or period. Approached in love rather than with the law, the question is no longer "What is permitted?" but rather "What does it mean to love my neighbor?" Approached in faith rather than considering works, the question ceases to be "What constitutes a breach of divine law in the sexual realm?" and becomes "What constitutes obedience to God as revealed in Jesus Christ?" Approached in the spirit rather than the letter of the law, the question ceases to be "What does the scripture demand?" and becomes "What word does the Spirit speak to the churches now in light of tradition, theology, psychology, genetics, anthropology and biology?"

Jesus once said, "Why don't you judge for yourselves what is right?" (Luke 12:57). This kind of freedom surprises us as Christians for we would much rather be told what to do.

Grace links us with a person, not just a mandate. It gives us the freedom to say yes. Don'ts become dos. When we "fall in love" with Christ, we learn to love his rules and regulations because they are his will for us. Christ comes to us as the one who is our relentless and compassionate "lover." He embraces us where we are and is continually committed to our health and well-being. The law, then, is internalized and our identity is no longer oppressed with a need to prove its innocence.

3. The life-giving filter invites us to a life of responsibility. When asked for his advice in response to the AIDS crisis, Dr. C. Everett Koop, the surgeon general of the

United States, responded simply, "Teach young people personal responsibility and self-respect." "That's it?" we cry. Our practical predicament is the nagging discomfort that a life-giving response (or grace) is not nice and neat. There is no Cliffs Notes book for moral choices, no page of easy-to-read instructions for all the choices along the way. The Christian gospel introduces us to a tender, compassionate and relentless lover who doesn't seem put off by our arrogance, self-indulgence or self-pity. And he announces the truth that we are loved and therefore free to live life in that light—free to say no to tyranny and free to say yes to self-respect, personal dignity, commitments and living responsibly.

The absence of a dictionary that details exact behavior for every moral circumstance need not mean that every moral choice brings with it the heaviness of moral tyranny, as if each choice is a win-or-lose proposition. Such is the predicament of the legalist. But win-or-lose propositions change the mood from responsibility to oppression, from the journey to the destination, from the freedom to risk and give to a heavy self-consciousness, from being other-focused to being self-focused.

Grace says we are free to proceed with life without a nervous glance over our shoulder. We're free to enjoy life because our identity is not dependent upon how we perform; therefore, we're free to be responsible.

Responsible for our choices. Responsible people own the choices they make. Both risk and responsibility can be taken because there is no obligation to an identity determined by some public opinion poll. There is no need to play life safe, measuring words and second-guessing choices. There is no need to treat life as a trial run, hoping that if we get our lines right, we can avoid any conflict in the real play.

Responsible for our actions. Responsible people are "wide awake" to what's going on around them, including people, feelings and circumstances. Too often, we charge through life like "a bull in a china shop," intent on carrying out our predetermined moral agenda. And we miss the signals of need, hurt and the ditches by the side of the road.

Responsible people know there is more to life and morality than being right.

Responsible for our reasons. Responsible people have no problem explaining themselves to others. If our identity is intact, we're free to own our choices. There is no need to point fingers. There is no need to practice a no-fault confession. We no longer have any innocence to protect. Hiding behind "what will they think" only encourages us to be victims of life. And responsible people are not victims, but gallant fighters.

▶ Living Responsibly in a Complex World

A life-giving response is an invitation to live responsibly. How do we translate this invitation to our specific situations? Are there some helpful tools for translation? Smedes offers a list of questions for the responsible person. Because of their benefit and their reflection of the life-giving filter, I will repeat the list and briefly expand on each question: [13]

Have I used discernment? I want to be right. And sometimes being right clashes with being moral. The issue here is not orthodoxy, but wisdom. When reality hurts, I want to avoid it. My pain can trick me into sorting out only that which fits comfortably into my own life. But there is more to making moral choices than making life fit. Morality is about people. Have I looked at the situation? at the people? at the circumstances? at the timing? Have I remembered that rules break but people tear?

Have I interpreted the question? It's true that a surface issue isn't always the real issue and a surface question isn't always the real question. Have I listened? Am I so intent at making a point, performing a duty or rescuing the day that I miss the true focus? Am I like the missionary who responded to a native's request for water by giving a sermon about the water of life? It's as if I walk through life handling every moral choice with a blunt object. And if my only tool were a hammer, every problem would be a nail. I have forgotten there is no prewritten script to determine how I do what I do.

Did my action fit the situation? Did I do what was appropriate in the unique situation that demanded a hard decision? I remember Dennis, a single parent who had custody of his handicapped teenage daughter. One day we received word that Dennis had been accused of raping his daughter and was being detained in the county jail. Dennis did not deny the charges and was ready to accept the penalty for his actions. Convinced of Dennis' repentance, a group from our church decided to raise money to post bail so Dennis could spend the months before his trial as a free man. The group asked if Dennis could participate in regular church activities. Others opposed this idea and suggested I tell Dennis' church class of his crime, as protection to the group. I almost consented, but then realized I would be sacrificing Dennis' dignity for my own moral uprightness. Rules are easy, but discernment is tough.

Does it support my commitments? If I am responsible, I will make and keep my commitments. I will also know when to break a bad commitment or one that was poorly made. A persistent theme in this book has been that morality is about investment in life: investment in people and investment in commitments. That's important because morality cannot be divorced from relationships, and "commitments are the backbone of human relationships . . . When we commit ourselves to people, we create an island of certainty for them in the ocean of life's swelling uncertainties. When everything else goes berserk and life seems to be falling apart at the seams, the people we know are given one certainty: We will be there with them. People can count on us when we make commitments and keep them."[14]

Some decisions are easier than others. Does having an affair jeopardize my commitment with my spouse? As a single person, does casual intercourse affect my commitment to my self-respect? But other decisions are not as easy. Is the marriage commitment violated if I become friends with a good-looking colleague of the opposite sex? Is the commitment to honesty violated if I withhold information from a previous relationship, knowing it would be damaging? Is commitment to a friendship violated if I share private information with a future employer for my friend's best interest?

Is the commitment to celibacy violated if I am in a relationship where intercourse is avoided, but as a couple we regularly enjoy mutual masturbation?

I want a yes or a no, a nice and neat morality. But yes or no is not the issue. The issue is wrestling with my commitments. When I pretend my struggles are easier than they are, I am avoiding responsibility to my commitment.

Have I used my imagination? Am I sacrificing people for the sake of rules? If morality is personal and relational, then moral choices require an element of creativity. The alternative is a predetermined script. Even the best rules can endorse action that makes moral people do the wrong thing. I must use my imagination to make sure those who are innocent don't suffer.

Am I willing to go public? Personal isolation only clouds intentionality. In secret, it's easier to give in to the mood, the urge or the moment. Temptation is testimony to the reality that it's easier to make healthy decisions when my desires are not aided by secrecy. "No one will know, so who will it hurt?" I ask, not really waiting for an answer. The question can be rephrased: "Am I choosing environments (and circumstances) in my relationships that are life-giving?" "Will my choices be healthier over lunch in broad daylight or in a candle-lit corner of a secluded restaurant?" "Will my choices be healthier if my spouse is a part of my friendship with an opposite-sex colleague or if the relationship is kept clandestine?" Of course, broad daylight hardly guarantees moral behavior, but responsible people know that a relationship probably isn't healthy if one has to lie or hide.

Am I willing to accept the consequences? Responsible people don't need to excuse themselves from the table of moral choices when it comes time to pay the bill, nor do they need to assume the role of martyr. I think of the story of Mike and Renee. Both in their late 20s, they had dated for about six months when they decided to end the relationship. "No future," they decided. Six weeks after the breakup, Renee discovered she was pregnant. She was shocked because the pregnancy obviously wasn't planned, and because she and Mike had had intercourse only once, and that during the final week of their dating relationship.

Faced with a moral dilemma, Renee and Mike began to sort through their options. They went back and forth but came to the realization that both abortion and adoption were out of the question. And, as far as they were concerned, so was marriage. But they did decide to pursue joint therapy. They chose to confront and walk through the anger, hurt, resentment and frustration that accompanied the news of the pregnancy. It was a tough road, but they continued. With the help of therapy, they realized they could commit to a relationship—a relationship of their own free choice—and together commit to raising their child. Four months after the baby's birth, the couple were married. A difficult choice for both people, but one that accepted and owned responsibility and the consequences.

Life-giving morality is about permission to live life fully, permission to see life as a journey, permission to hear the music, permission to paint a picture and permission to fall in love with the Lawgiver who has already fallen in love with you. To the one who has heard this voice of grace comes the freedom to choose life.

I close with a story from Brennan Manning. "A woman came to see a priest and she said, 'Would you come and pray with my daddy? He's dying of cancer and he wants to die at home.' The priest went to the house and, when he walked into the man's room, he saw the man lying on the bed with an empty chair beside the bed. The priest asked the man if someone had been visiting. The man replied, 'Oh, let me tell you about that chair. I've never told anyone this—not even my daughter. I hope you don't think I'm weird, but all of my life I have never known how to pray. I've read books on prayer, heard talks on prayer, but nothing ever worked. Then, a friend told me that prayer was like a conversation with Jesus. He suggested that I put a chair in front of me, imagine Jesus sitting in the chair, and talk to Him. Since that day, I've never had any difficulty praying. I hope you don't think I am off-the-wall.' The priest assured the man that there was nothing weird about praying to Jesus in a chair. The priest anointed the man and left. Two days later, the daughter called to say that her father had just died. The priest asked, 'Did he die peaceful-ly?' She replied, 'I left him at 2:00 this afternoon. He had a smile on his face when I walked out the door. He even told me one of his corny jokes. When I returned at 3:30, he was dead. One curious thing, though—his head was resting not on the bed, but on an empty chair beside his bed.' To this man, Jesus was an intimate friend, and so he died with his friend. All changes, all growth, all improvements in the quality of our lives flow out of our vision of God. And when our vision of God is one of a God of relentless ten-derness, we ultimately become tender ourselves."[15]

▶ Discussion Questions

1. "Christian faith is not in the ethics business at all, but in the identity business . . . My identity has little to do with my points earned or squandered" (page 153). If these statements are true, how do they affect you and your rela-tionship with God? with others?

2. The life-giving approach is a gift of grace; it means we can live life "from" acceptance rather than "for" ac-ceptance (page 154). What is the difference? How does that difference affect your life?

3. In what ways does the fact that our identity is intact in the hands of a faithful God (page 155) impact your deci-sion-making?

4. How does the life-giving approach change your focus from don'ts to dos (pages 157-158)? Think of a personal il-lustration or an example to illustrate this new focus.

5. Read the responsibility questions again (pages 160-163). Choose the question that has been most helpful to you in a practical way.

6. How does the story by Brennan Manning reflect the life-giving approach (pages 163-164)? Imagine Jesus sitting in a chair next to you. What expectations of Jesus would you have in a meeting with him? What expectations of yourself would you have for this meeting? Would this meeting be life-giving for you? Explain. You may want to write about your own life-giving experience. Share your story with someone you trust.

►CHAPTER 11

Objections, You Say?

"Morality is the need to make right choices. Forgiveness is the freedom to make wrong choices."—Lewis Smedes[1]

"Well?" asked the small, blond woman with the dancing brown eyes. She had listened intently through the entire workshop from her front row seat. I had just finished my final lecture in a series on sex and choices. The lecture was on grace and life-giving decision-making.

"Well, what?" I responded.

"Well, what's your answer about sex? What do you really think?" She wanted closure.

I had no answer for her then, and I still don't. There is no single sentence or paragraph that could encapsulate the entire issue, make sense out of the incongruity we feel, heal our woundedness, assuage our guilt, recognize and applaud our efforts and assure us that life will be as easy as the life of our dreams. Besides, if her question were about intercourse, what the Bible has to say about genital behavior and commitment is clear enough. But I'm convinced there's more at stake here.

You see, grace makes all of us uncomfortable. It seems we would rather read a "How, When and Where Guide to One's Genitals." But grace dares to say that the issue of sex and the choices we make is more comprehensive than our genitals, our moral credentials, our acquired technique, our correct theology, our selfish shortcomings and our answers.

Grace—or the life-giving choice—is about the permission and freedom to live as a human being, fully alive and whole. And that's not possible if we continue to equate our wholeness, or capacity to be human, with morality and religion. What we are saying is that Christianity isn't really interested in the morality business. "Ethics tells you what you ought and ought not to do in order to be recognizably and acceptably human. Christianity tells you about a God who takes unrecognizable and unacceptable human beings and recognizes and accepts them in Jesus, whether or not they happen to have done what they ought to have done."[2] My responses to an individual's questions about specific sexual behaviors are secondary at best. Grace refocuses us on the primary issues—how the symbols of Christian faith allow us to see more clearly the foundation of our identity and illumine a path in a world filled with ambiguity and confusion.

The issues are hardly resolved, but as you recall, that was never our intention. Sexuality is always a relational issue, and dialogue is essential. So, let's do just that. Here is my response to some of the objections or concerns I have heard expressed after my workshops.

1. "Isn't the life-giving approach to moral choices situational?" The answer is yes. As Robert Capon says, "Morality, [by] its very nature, must be concerned with norms, with standards; whereas grace, by definition, is concerned with persons."[3] I understand the fear here. The idea of grace and personal responsibility is good, but we don't want this idea to get out of hand. And it sounds too similar to narcissism, like some kind of "situational ethics."

But the Bible does not bring closure to our moral lives. Much is left open and gray—choices that will be dictated by responsibility. Two concerns are at work here. The first is a personal concern. We may not be aware of it or it may be subconscious; but it is there nonetheless. We are afraid of losing control of our dark side. Some of us have worked hard at being in control and presenting an impenetrable facade. What will happen now that we have been given the freedom to choose? After being "slaves to a script" for so long, what will we do now with our freedom?

Our second concern is about others, those for whom we take responsibility. Our need for control extends to those around us. Perhaps we want to convince ourselves that if we can control others, we will not be so concerned about our own internal contradictions—those surprising parts of our inner and emotional life that we work so hard to repress.

The life-giving approach means getting dirty—getting down in the trenches of real life with real people. Moral choices are actually people issues. Jesus was life-giving because he didn't see crowds or scripts; he saw individuals, faces, concerns and circumstances. He refused to strip people of their dignity by reducing their plight to answers on a true-false test.

2. "If I teach the life-giving approach, won't people take advantage and interpret it as license?" So what else is new? It's our nature to take advantage. We talked earlier in the book about our addictive natures. We talked about how we love things and use people, how we seek relief in the temporary, how we sacrifice what is best for what is immediate. Even our facade as a moralist reveals its true nature as we race up and down the line looking for loopholes. We are notorious for taking advantage of and using the system.

In a recent ad for motorcycles, the question was explicit: "What are you waiting for—permission?" The ad reduced the issue to a behavioral dilemma: to buy or not to buy. People are reduced to victims. As mindless consumers, we wait for the media gods to tell us what we need and give us permission to "go for it." The church has a tendency to treat the issue of moral choices the same way. We protect the flock by eliminating the options.

"But didn't you give people license in your talk?" one concerned church leader asked.

I understand from where the question comes. I just don't believe that adults have been waiting all their lives for some speaker (or preacher or author) to give them permission to engage in a behavior that they may believe is wrong but have perhaps secretly wished to do. They hardly need me, or anyone else for that matter, for permission. And even so, the reality of permission hardly nullifies grace.

He was 30 years old, and his question was blunt and to the point. "Can we do it?"

"Can you do what?" I asked.

"Can my girlfriend and I have sex as long as we're committed to each other?" he asked, obviously in a hurry for his answer. (Again he was equating sex with intercourse only.)

"If you mean 'can' as in, 'Is it an option?' the answer is yes," was my response. "If you want to know whether you're free to choose whatever behavior you want, the answer is yes. If you want to know whether God will change his opinion about you, the answer is no. You're free to choose. You're free to invest in the sanctity of life, and you're free to fail."

Free to choose and free to fail—because we are loved. "All Jesus did was announce the truth of that and tell you it would make you free. It was admittedly a dangerous thing to do. You *are* a menace. But he did it, and therefore, menace or not, here you stand, uncondemned, forever, *now.* What are you going to do with your freedom?"[4]

Yes, I guess I do give you license. License to believe you are loved and license to fall in love with the one who loves you.

But wait a minute. If a certain behavior is wrong, doesn't the church have an obligation to tell people so? Capon answers: "Not, I think, at the price of giving the world the impression that the Church's main business is sin-prevention. God in Jesus didn't prevent sin, He forgave it. If the Church wants to represent Him, it shouldn't go around misrepresenting His methods. It should instead busy itself with the twin jobs of forgiving sinners and healing the sick with, in short, the Gospel work of raising the dead."[5] The world is not a collection of good listeners waiting for the right advice to come along.

Our job is not to keep people in line. Our job is to repeat the truth of the good news. I heard a story about a Texas woman who had five sons. They were grown boys, ranging from their teens to their early 20s. And they were hellions, with quite a reputation for their ability to party and get into trouble. Nonetheless, this mother always referred to her boys as "my sons, the saints." Others around her would remind her of her boys' actions by saying things like "You mean the saints who just tore up the county courthouse?" "Oh," she would reply, "they just forgot who they were!"

That's good theology, and it's good understanding about the foundational issue regarding sex and the moral choices we make. Our identity is at stake. Lack of faith in ourselves results from a loss of memory. We have forgotten who really owns us. We have forgotten that God loves us— you and me—for no good reason at all.

Still unsure? Doesn't that mother's attitude give continued license to a negative lifestyle? Again, we confuse grace with permission. I conduct a workshop on "Beginning Again" that expands upon life after divorce. Many churches refuse to offer such a course, arguing that it encourages divorce. That's like saying that if you set up a fire department, you encourage people to set fires. No doubt there will always be pyromaniacs in addition to a good number of careless buffoons, but that hardly nullifies grace. It's the pyromaniacs who lose, not grace. When we fail to respond to the fullness of life, "we do not simply get our selves in dutch; rather, we fail to become ourselves at all."[6]

3. "But there is still no real measurement for right and wrong." I know I stand to ruffle a lot of feathers. Many of you still see me as the moral policeman, and you're waiting for an answer. Can we or can't we? A man in Orlando literally cornered me after a talk. "Okay," he said

intently, "I've listened to your talk. I've read as many books as I can get my hands on. But now it's just you and me. And I want your answer on sex. Don't beat around the bush anymore!"

I still did not answer his question. Why? Because he really didn't want an answer. He wanted to be set free from the responsibility that comes with making personal choices. He wanted to remain a victim. When we can implicate a moral policeman in our choices, we can assume the role of victim. Someone else will take responsibility for our choices if we can say, "The minister (or the workshop leader) told me so."

Beating around the bush, you say? Backing away from biblical standards? Promoting license? I'm in trouble already. It's not that the Bible doesn't talk about fornication or the connection between intercourse and marriage. It definitely does. But answering that question does not resolve the issue. The issue is far more fundamental. You see, if I say yes, people for the most part—both singles and marrieds—are inwardly glad, but outwardly they are righteously indignant. "How could he be so blatantly liberal?" People are looking for permission (or at least a release from the urges of their dark side) or a target for moral projection. And I will not provide either because both remove us from responsibility. If I say no, it's seen as the religious party line. People merely shrug their shoulders and say: "See there. I told you what he'd say. He's no help. He just doesn't understand."

So, does not answering the question mean I am avoiding the issue? I think not. It means I am changing the focus of the issue. The issue now is our personal responsibility and its consequences. Does that mean a "roll in the hay" will bring down lightning and the judgment of God? I don't think so. And contrary to some teaching, I don't think it will scar you for life. On the other hand, you can't give yourself away without some consequences—like learning to live with the law of diminished returns. It's only in the fairy tale world of television that you can "have your cake and eat it too."

"But wait! You've given us no standards!" On the contrary. Grace (the life-giving approach) is a much more encompassing standard than legalism, and at the same time, far more liberating than narcissism. We want a standard that will judge whether or not we receive merit points for hitting the right notes. We're willing to sacrifice integrity for achievement (or uprightness), and character (being) for conduct (doing). Public opinion becomes more important than personal dignity. In the end, we use people for our moral protection.

The standard of grace says merit points no longer matter. There is no moral contest. Our identity is no longer in limbo, pending some crowd-pleasing, moral high-wire act. Grace says our identity is already intact. It says: "Because my own life has worth and dignity, I can treat others in the same way. I don't need to manipulate others or use anyone to prove anything."

According to the gospel, grace has already offered us a position on life's winning team. "Thus [the] church is not one more place for [us] to compete and get a performance rating. Like a victorious locker room, [the] church is a place [for us] to exult, to give thanks, to celebrate the great news that all is forgiven, that God is love, that victory is certain."[7]

4. "Isn't the life-giving approach hard to teach?"
Yes. The approach is not only hard to teach, but hard to hear because we would much rather be comfortable than grow. Control and closure are important to our needs for comfort, both as teachers and as disciples. We want our lives based on logical equations and our identities based on moral performances that fulfill specific requirements. It seems that "you can get people to buy acceptance after their sins are under control, or only when their disasters have been forestalled by proper behavior."[8]

Looking good is the enticement of our generation, the lure of our selfishness. Life-giving morality is difficult to teach because it doesn't reward those who have spent their lives and energies trying to look good. From the "I'm not such a bad guy" narcissist in us to the "I'm not as bad as the backslider" legalist in us, we focus on keeping our own reputations clean.

The life-giving approach is hard to teach and hear because the gospel has little to do with reputations—clean or otherwise. To the heart set on receiving affirmation for deeds done or deeds avoided, the gospel message of grace is a letdown. Why? Because in reality any efforts we make are all destined to fail—from our excursions into the world of absolute freedom to our hikes to the top of the mountain where we are king. The gospel isn't looking for good guys, self-appointed kings or successful and disciplined achievers. The gospel is looking for people who know they aren't any of those things. Freedom actually begins with a profound awareness that we are, in and of ourselves, powerless, and that life, if it is anything, is a free and gracious gift.

We've come full circle. We began this book with the realization that sexuality and moral choices could not be reduced to behavioral issues. And we come back to that same emphasis. Morality and sexuality are, always have been and always will be, identity issues. Fullness of life begins when we know we are unconditionally and freely loved. We are free when we can begin to slowly dismantle the armor we've accumulated to keep life from hurting us, when we begin to slowly tear up the moral score cards that we have worked so hard to master, and when we are no longer treated as objects or rungs on others' ladders to happiness.

I no longer need to run from my dark side, justify my sinfulness, rationalize my fault lines, repress my irrational nature, be embarrassed by my weaknesses, or brag about my moral accomplishments. I can own me—all of me— and I can confess. I can be loved and healed only because I recognize that I am in need. Easy? Hardly. But the ideal of life-giving choices based on grace has not been tried and found wanting; it has been found difficult and not tried. So "do not preach us grace . . . Give us something, anything; but spare us the indignity of this indiscriminate acceptance."9

Where do we go from here? I have two recommendations. Number one, I give you permission to let God fall in love with you. Begin to see the persistent, relentless and tender love of God. Be awakened to an overwhelming sense of a personal, holy, compassionate God. Understand that when you allow yourself to receive such love, you begin to fall in love with the giver. The issue with morality is not permission to do right or wrong; the issue is becoming new people and becoming alive.

Because of the cross, we don't have to or got to or ought to or should—we *want* to change, because we know how deeply we are loved. The secret is not to fight sin, but to embrace Jesus. All of us have been given permission to live life with "Amazing Grace" as our theme song. And if we think it's essential to be religious or churched to begin this process, we've missed the point.

Number two, because of number one, I encourage you to take more risks. Know that your identity is intact in the hands of a faithful God and you are free to fail. Too many of us live our moral lives with a calculator and a behavioral almanac. I agree with Smedes: "Dare to be wrong! Risk it! With forgiveness you discover that being wrong is not all that bad. No wrong choice you make can persuade God to love you less. Believe this and you will have new courage to make choices even when you are not sure they will be the right ones to make. [Have the] courage to fail."[10]

I am reminded of the story of the late Artur Rubinstein who was often accused of playing the wrong notes. When one critic made a particular issue of these lapses by the maestro, another critic replied, "Yes, but what wrong notes!"

▶ **Discussion Questions**

1. "Christianity isn't really interested in the morality business" (page 168). What does this statement mean to you? How does this concept affect you personally?

2. "The life-giving approach to moral choices is situational" (pages 168-169). How do you feel about this statement? What is your greatest concern about this approach?

3. "People will take advantage of the life-giving approach and interpret it as license" (pages 169-171). This fear has been expressed by numerous individuals. How did the author respond? What did you think of his response? Would you be inclined to take advantage of the life-giving approach? Why or why not?

4. Some argue that, with the life-giving approach to morality, there is no standard (pages 171-173). Do you agree or disagree? Explain the role of grace within the life-giving approach.

5. What makes life-giving decision-making difficult to teach (pages 173-174)? List your concerns about the life-giving approach and discuss them with a friend. Don't expect all your questions to be answered or all your struggles to be resolved. You certainly won't agree with your friend on every point, but continue to meet and support one another in your struggles.

►SECTION FOUR:

Relationship Dynamics

►
___

Introduction

*I*f morality is relational, then community is essential to health. We do a disservice to ourselves—and to our discussions—when we assume we can approach the subject of sexuality as isolated units, as if choice-making is most effective in a vacuum. Coupled with the erroneous assumption that sexual morality is strictly behavioral, we come to the decision-making process in hopes that the decision will be a left-brain activity, a predicament that can be resolved with sufficient knowledge or information. We tend to emphasize the cognitive, where black and white, right and wrong, and correct answers are more important than health.

In the church we fan the flames of this rugged individualism by advocating a "just me and Jesus" theology. The result is unfortunate. Striving to prove our worthiness as individual players, we see vulnerability as a threat. We work to strengthen our self-discipline, believing we can handle it on our own—whether it be the struggle of sexual issues or just life in general. And the fact that we're not above the struggle only causes us to repress our real feelings in favor of those that are more acceptable.

It's a simple fact: We cannot handle life on our own. Self-sufficiency is our preference, but we need friends. Some of us attempt to avoid that need by busily accumulating large numbers of friends. We create the illusion that we are open, vulnerable and relational, while in reality we are using the infrequency and superficiality of many relationships to hide, even from ourselves. For when we are intimate with everyone, we are intimate with no one.

All of us need friends. We need both individual relationships and a group of friends that provide a support structure. How do these two relationships differ?

I like Merle Shain's definition. She says, "Friends are people who help you be more yourself, more the person you are intended to be, and it is possible that without them we don't recognize ourselves, or grow to be what it is in us to be."[1] When I am thinking clearly, I know that's what I need—someone to remind me that I approach life with the blinders of my own pain, concerns and anxieties. I need someone who will remind me that the world is bigger than who I am and what I am afraid of, that I am not a rock or an island, and that life is not easier from the vantage point of a fortress. Such truths I easily forget without a friend.

With a friend I begin to regain perspective about what is really important in my life. I need someone to remind me I am not a discardable commodity like I feel during those times when I wallow in my guilt and these times when I say, "If only . . ." I need someone to remind me I'm not invulnerable to the pain and loneliness of being human, to the consequences of bad decisions or to the anxiety that comes from wanting to be above it all.

But knowing I need a friend isn't always enough. I can easily assume the role of victim by waiting for some friend to appear and begin his or her appointed role. Unfortunately, it doesn't work that way. To gain a friend, I must be a friend. And that's not easy because it means risking. Most of us have already risked and lost once too often. So the thought of risking again is greeted with reluctance and a new layer of defense.

Sometimes I avoid the vulnerability of risking by assuming the role of the rescuer and fixing those around me. The issue is control. But being a friend and having a friend means receiving. And that is difficult because it means losing control. It means the relationship is more important than any projection of power, superiority, control, rightness or wrongness.

Listen again to Shain: "The job of a friend is not to decide what should be done, not to run interference or pick up the slack. The job of a friend is to understand, and to supply energy and hope, and in doing so to keep those they value on their feet a little longer, so that they can fight another round and grow stronger in themselves."[2]

Support groups or covenant groups are extensions of this friendship process. These gatherings are committed to personal and mutual health. Their purpose is focus and affirmation. Support groups, however, are not just fun gatherings; they are intentional. A support group is a group of three to 12 people (it can go higher, but the level of communication is impaired after 12). The group meets regularly—at least twice a month—at a set time for the purpose of nurturing and encouraging one another in specific areas of personal and spiritual growth. Our culture, with its emphasis upon individualism, sees support groups as optional behavior at best. In the church we see the value of support groups, but invariably we ask, "Aren't they primarily for people with problems?"

I hardly wish to add support groups to the existing long list of mandated behaviors, as if a group is another obligation necessary for our acceptance. On the other hand, I would be remiss if I didn't point to the danger of isolation. Support groups are important in reminding us of our identity—a place where we don't need to perform or give in to the equal tyranny of our selfishness. It's a place where we don't run from ambiguity, where we feel no need to squelch doubt or run from pain or our shadow side. It's a place where we can celebrate healthy choices and heal wounds that come from unhealthy choices. The support group can be a channel where God's grace becomes real.

How do such groups begin? Maybe you can begin one where you are. It's a matter of asking. Start with a group of three to five people. Set aside a time every week (or every other week) to meet in a comfortable setting. Agree on a purpose and agenda, and establish a time frame—whether it be six weeks or six months.

Being a part of a support group isn't always easy. The

success of a group is dependent upon healthy group communication. So, as a helpful tool, here's a list of effective ideas to support group dynamics.

▶ Effective Ways to Support Group Dynamics

1. Use "I" language instead of "you," "he," "she" or "they" language. It's important to make your statements personal.

2. Use "I feel" statements rather than "I think" statements. Focus on individual feelings rather than opinions and advice.

3. Keep everything confidential. Don't see the group as an opportunity for gossip.

4. Express your emotions. Encourage other group members to share their feelings of sadness, anger, badness or hope.

5. Allow periods of silence. Sometimes people need time to think as well as talk.

6. Encourage humor. When people can laugh at themselves, it makes it easier to accept imperfection.

7. Take special care not to spiritualize everything. When there is an answer or closure on every discussion, people soon learn it's not okay to continue the struggle.

8. When conflict of opinion or differences occur, encourage group members to talk about them. Remind the group it's not always necessary to agree.

9. Encourage other members of the group. Take care to affirm one another for honest sharing or recognizing a need.

10. Always start and end on time.

When group members consciously employ these effective ideas for group dynamics, they can help one another maintain honest relationships as they struggle together to support one another in their efforts.

Understanding our sexuality begins in community with others. The dynamics of relationships offer not only understanding but also healing and support if we are willing to risk our struggles. As we join others in this journey toward wholeness, we encourage one another in our mistakes and celebrate these relationships that help us become who we are created to be.

►CHAPTER 1 2

Implications for the Journey

> *"The essence of wisdom about sex is to understand that we are really in trouble when we think we have figured out the answers."*—Andrew Greeley[1]

We've been invited on a journey. And like all journeys, what you pack is important. If you're like me, there's a tendency to pack far too much. We need permission, especially in this area of sexuality, to travel lighter. We want a formula. We secretly hope that sooner or later some author will give us the answers. Then we can be on our way, armed with the assurance that such answers will help us avoid the ambiguity of real-life choices.

But the sexuality issue cannot be resolved once and for all. We need to concern ourselves not where we arrive, but with the direction we're going. And while we hope to arm ourselves against the ambiguity of real-life drama with resolutions and quick-fix pieces of advice, we soon find ourselves sent back into the world with its struggles and confusion. At this point we realize hope is not found in solutions or catch phrases, but in the permission to embrace the journey itself. And how is that done? It's done with responsible choices that lend themselves to health. I recommend packing the following choices for the journey.

1. Learn and teach the life-giving approach and the principles of grace, not just rules. Our morality is not determined by some detached intellectual judgment. It's not enough for us to make pronouncements regarding some laundry list of behaviors. Why? Because morality is about who we are, not just what we do. Moral choices are not academic exercises; they are personal. And as we've said, there is no predetermined script. Morality is about what it means to be human. It is about emotional investment in life, relationships, commitments and health. It means receiving permission to take a look at ourselves— both the good and bad.

Every moral choice is therefore an identity issue. We begin with the foundation of our identity. Recognizing who (or what) owns us determines the choices we make. It will not do, then, for us to be behaviorists—reducing life and morality to a list and defining our identity by the sum of the behavioral parts. Like the Pharisees, we have to learn that there's more to life than answering all the questions right. For sex is more than intercourse, and the issue of moral choices about sex is bigger than what we do with our genitals.

As Christians, we are called to be prophets to one another. In a moving story from the New Testament, a woman of questionable reputation anoints Jesus with an expensive perfume. The religious leaders and disciples are outraged and ask questions such as "How could you allow this, Jesus? Isn't this a sheer waste of money? Do you know who this woman is?" The religious leaders wanted to reduce the woman's identity to the sum of her behavioral parts—a wasteful, rude prostitute—and technically, they were right. But Jesus assumed the role of prophet to those around him. He did not look at things as they were, but the way they could become. So he responded: "She has done a beautiful thing to me . . . Wherever the gospel is preached throughout the world, what she has done will also be told, in memory of her" (Mark 14:6, 9). Jesus gave her a new identity. Before he judged her as right or wrong, he deemed her loved—worthy, valuable, a child of dignity. He gave her permission to believe that her identity was more than the sum of the parts.

This life-giving approach isn't easy to teach; and it's definitely not easy to practice. For example, after doing a workshop for ministers on the issue of life-giving morality for young adults, there was a good deal of discomfort. "But you have no rights and wrongs with your system," said one leader. Another asked: "What if they still choose to go to bed with each other? How do we let them know this is wrong?"

I understood their questions, but they missed the point. My concern as a minister or leader is not to keep young adults out of bed or away from sex. With enough guilt, I could lead a group of people to do all the right things for all the wrong reasons. (Pharisaism is what Jesus called it; and it kills like cancer.) I prefer to offer young adults a place where they can be honest about the gift of their God-given sexuality. I want to teach them and myself how to receive a love from God that is not based on performance, technique or righteous limitations. If we honestly believe in God's unconditional love, that love will begin to own us and will affect our decisions. As was quoted in Chapter 10, "Jesus evidently didn't want people to neurotically concentrate on 'not sinning,' but rather to focus on loving God and people."[2]

Our focus must be on wholeness, nurture and health, not just for single people, but for everyone. Marriage doesn't guarantee that our sexual behaviors are life-giving. Both singles and marrieds are called to be personally responsible. "Young adult ministry at its best is an environment that nurtures personal responsibility. How do we face the pressure of our supersexed generation? We slowly learn to let God love us. Legalistic environments only reinforce the performance mentality that young adults live with daily in the world they encounter. The church must be different."[3]

2. Give up your moral policeman badge. Because I was a behaviorist—seeing life as a contest, seeing morality as a list, seeing the Christian faith as a test—becoming a moral policeman was a convenient way to cover up my own insecurities. I assumed I could control life by controlling those around me. By placing myself in such a position of power, I felt exempt from the need to examine my own vulnerability, weaknesses and obsessions. I failed to see that my moral policeman badge was a crutch. I was struggling to maintain my identity, my ability to be a strong leader. I said my desire was to make my group morally pure, but the real reason was hidden. I wanted the group to be a good reflection on my reputation. The group members were no longer people, but points on my resume. This style is obsessive, and the irony is that it ultimately objectifies evil, treating it as though it were something foreign to ourselves, something that could be avoided like a disease if only we would stay away from it.

Consequently, our temptation is to remove the freedom and construct a system where the person is not allowed to sin. The message to those around us is loud and clear: "You are not to be trusted." "This brings persons to undervalue themselves and to mistrust their own judgment, to throw away, in other words, the very aspects of their personality through which they define their moral presence in life."[4] Success is more than just not failing.

Invariably, such a message is a projection of our own inner struggle and the difficulty we have in self-trust. We react by making life manageable. But if God is who he says he is, then we can learn to trust people to make changes. We are not the change agent in people's lives. If God is who he says he is, then we don't need to trick people into change by using behavioral techniques, manipulating with guilt or providing heavy-handed recommendations. If God is who he says he is, we can give up our need to rescue others or our personal need to feel continually offended by their insensibilities. If God is who he says he is, then we can trust him to shower other people with his love and we can become agents of that message.

Jesus never took away the freedom to fail. He didn't treat his disciples as adolescents. He knew that "morality only arises where there is enough elbowroom in which to look around and make decisions" and that "morality grows when people give themselves permission to live."[5] He let them own the responsibility and consequences for their choices and was there for them when they were ready to return.

3. Become part of a support structure, and encourage others to do the same. We don't need more insights, admonition or hellfire. Like alcoholics, we rarely respond to lectures on what we should or should not do. But unlike alcoholics, we fail to realize how much we need people. We need a place like Alcoholics Anonymous where our identity can find a solid foundation of love, respect, support and accountability. Teaching has never changed moral behavior. Real change can only happen internally, personally and individually. But it can happen only when we know we are in need. We must remind ourselves that Christianity is not a moral discovery for those who have arrived, but is a gift to those who know they haven't arrived and are still struggling with what it means to be human.

To be healthy is a daily choice. It cannot be circumvented by repression (for not to choose is to choose), busyness or the right answers. It's a choice that begins with the daily acknowledgment of our neediness and the reality that in the area of sexuality none of us need to pretend that we have our act together. Andrew Greeley provides us a way to acknowledge this continuing choice in what he calls the "Five Rules for Living With Sexual Hunger":[6]

▶ Five Rules for Living With Sexual Hunger

1. We must accept the tremendous power of our sexuality and acknowledge the weakness and inadequacy of our control over that power.

2. We must accept the fact that our sexuality flows in many strange eddies and currents and can be diverted down dark, hateful and punitive streams.

3. We must accept the fact that the same ill-controlled

and frequently deceptive power that we experience also exists in everyone else.

4. We must accept the fact that casual attitudes, simple formulae, easy answers and magic techniques are inadequate responses to the fearsome power of sex.

5. We must accept the fact that whatever our sexual posture (married or celibate), hard work and constant effort at focusing energies are necessary for both healthy relationships with members of the other sex and for the diversion of our excess sexual energies into constructive and creative activities.

That's why we need each other. Because none of us is complete in isolation. Because we have lousy memories about who really owns us. Because we have forgotten that our identity—both the dark side and the light—is intact in the hands of a faithful God. Because we no longer need to repeat self-destructive behaviors or prove our worth by accumulating points on the self-discipline scale of 1 to 10, or hand our identity over to another for approval and reassurance. Isolation is the enemy. We no longer need to pretend we are the solitary hero—fighting all odds and standing alone. We need to join with fellow journeyers and strugglers for perspective, support and accountability.

So I would like to add a sixth rule to Greeley's list.

6. We must accept the fact that we are incomplete people in a broken world, and we cannot make it alone.

4. Practice the reality of forgiveness. Here we begin with the truth that forgiveness is for me. It means that I recognize I don't have the ability to make myself whole again. I receive this gift through confession, through giving control back to God. When I practice the reality of forgiveness, I let God tell me that my identity and self-worth are bigger than my need to perform, my need to point a finger, my need to feel self-pity or my need to define myself by my failure. To be forgiven is to be set free! I don't need to be excused, nor do I always need to defend myself or wish that life were more fair. Forgiveness is God's way of telling me that I don't need to continue such behaviors to get his attention.

Forgiveness means being overwhelmed by a God who is crazy enough to want to be our friend. We receive forgiveness through confession and repentance, when we own our choices and behaviors and recognize their consequences.

Not all repentance, however, is healthy. Meister Eckhart, the 13th century German mystic, speaks of the two kinds of repentance: one "of time" and the other "divine."[7] The one of time—or of our natural senses—always leads to self-pity, a self-loathing that doesn't encourage sorrow, but despair. With this type of repentance there is no progress, no movement, no hope; only regret. Divine repentance, however, is the true sorrow in which individuals acknowledge their brokenness and lift themselves up to God. This acknowledgment and consequent dependence on God is based on the confidence and security that God's hands are loving.

C.S. Lewis writes: "Ask for God's help . . . After each failure, ask forgiveness, pick yourself up, and try again. Very often what God first helps us towards is not the virtue itself but just this power of always trying again. For however important chastity (or courage, or truthfulness, or any other virtue) may be, this process trains us in habits of the soul . . . It cures our illusions about ourselves and teaches us to depend on God."[8]

But sometimes we prefer to punish ourselves by carrying out our self-fulfilling prophecies that we are unlovable, worthless failures. In an ironic twist, it maintains our illusion of control. And, in the same way, we prefer to punish those around us by withholding forgiveness or waiting for some restitution. But forgiveness is not an equation or a release from guilt in exchange for an intent to perform properly. We're waiting for someone to say to us—just like we say to God—"I promise. I'll never do it again!" Real forgiveness is release, regardless of such a promise. It is God saying to us: "I release you from my need to punish you. I release you from your need to be defined by self-destruction. I release you to know that your identity is bigger than the sum of your behaviors." It is our saying to one another: "I give up my right to make you pay. I give up my right to exact a pound of flesh. I give up my right to prove that life must be fair. I give up my right to hold you liable for your past."

Unconditional acceptance is a frightening thought. What if people take advantage of forgiveness? What if people flaunt their freedom? It is frightening because it means receiving without any ability to repay.

5. Encourage commitment. Life does eventually clash with our expectations, which are nurtured by Madison Avenue and give us a sense of entitlement, a "right" to be happy. "The hardest lesson for this generation seems to be this: Choice is limited. You cannot do everything and be everything in one life."9

One way we teach commitment is by modeling. Commitment is modeled by offering effective boundaries. We must learn how to effectively say no and no longer rescue those who are trying to grow. Commitment means that our churches must become places that give away responsibility. It's one thing to watch and complain about the irresponsible and non-committed young adults in the group or church. It's another to begin giving away doses of responsibility. When we rescue people from responsibility by not letting them fail or set up an environment where people are not allowed to fail, we become moral policemen. We don't allow the church to be a place where people can think about their sexuality and struggle and choose. (As one pastor said: "Oh, we never have to deal with the issue of sex outside of marriage. It never happens here." Translation: "No one is allowed to talk about it here.")

Every commandment has a context. There is always a why to match the what. Yes, the Bible teaches that genital sex is to be practiced in a marital—or committed—context, and we don't need to manipulate biblical texts to see otherwise. But that is hardly the issue. The issue is commitment. And commitment focuses on the way we treat ourselves and other people. It means creating an environment where we nurture self-respect.

We need to create an environment where the emphasis

is not on success or failure, but on faithfulness—the art of simply trying. We need an environment where we practice honesty without threatening punishment if someone really tells the truth. We need an environment that understands that the issue of commitment is not confined to genital behavior, but spills over into the way we deal with our eating obsessions and our money. We also need an environment that willingly confronts our desire to gossip (our need to protect our reputations at others' expense) with as much energy as is spent on the issue of sexuality.

6. *Teach and learn a gracious reality.* When we fail to understand the context of a gracious reality, our natural desires lead to frustration because life always seems unfair. A gracious reality allows us to live with ambiguity. Why? Because ultimately, God is trustworthy. If in our minds we picture God as a capricious and arbitrary cosmic bookkeeper, then life becomes a relentless task. Risks are no longer worth taking, for the price of failure is too high. Love is for the lucky and the strong. We opt for security and look at ambiguity as the enemy. Life becomes a win-or-lose proposition in which being right is more important than being real.

But if reality is gracious—because God is ultimately gracious—then it is possible to take the risk of being fully alive. We can embrace life—dandelions and all. We can see God incognito in the struggle and the ordinariness of the journey. We can believe it's okay to choose, without guaranteeing the moral score of the outcome. We can experience love that's for the fighters—those people who try and try again. We can accept the fact that nothing can be gained by sacrificing reality for rightness.

When we believe that reality is built on grace, how do we respond? Listen again to Robert Capon: "Your part in it is just to make yourself available . . . Be open to your lover [God] who . . . started this whole affair. And your attendance upon him can include literally everything you do because he has accepted it all in the Beloved: all good acts because they are vindicated in him; all rotten acts because they are reconciled in him; and even all religious acts because, in him, they have ceased to be transactions and become celebrations of something already accomplished."[10] If this is true, it means we can now talk to God about our sexuality and the choices we make. We can bring him into the discussion. There is no need to cower at the mention of his name. He's not a spy from the other team.

It's difficult to bring God into the discussion because we're afraid we must promise never to fail again, as if God is waiting for some verbal pay back for his grace toward us. But God doesn't ask for such a promise. We let our pride get in the way—that inability to let another be our friend, that inability to need another. And we keep pushing God away. "We'll do it on our own," we say. "We'll ask for his presence when we have a good enough report card to impress him."

Fortunately, it's not what we continue to believe about God that's important here, but what he continues to believe about us. And he . . . well, he loves us for no good reason. He wants to be our friend, and he doesn't quit, whether we like it or not.

Case Studies

*F*ollowing are seven case studies. They're taken from real situations, so the names have been changed. Why include case studies in a book on sexuality? Because it gives us a chance to look at the stories of real people, real faces, real questions and real struggles. Moral choices are no longer nice and neat. Some of these stories may mirror our own lives by reflecting our own complexity, confusion and need for hope.

The case studies are to be used for group dialogue. They can be used in a class, workshop or home study group. Groups should be no larger than five people. The group's task is to read an individual's case and then assume the position of pastor, counselor, parent or concerned friend. The person in the case has come to you for counseling. What do you say to this person? What advice do you have? How do you help this person resolve the dilemma? What is your role in his or her resolution of this problem?

I recommend role playing: Set aside 30 minutes. Group members play the role of the people represented in the case study. One group member assumes the role of a "legalist" counselor or friend. After 10 minutes, another group member role plays the "narcissist" counselor or friend. After 10 more minutes, a third group member role plays a "life-giving" counselor or friend. Others in the group observe.

After all three counselors or friends have had their say, discuss what you observed. Were the approaches different? What did you expect each counselor or friend to say? What do you agree or disagree with? How did each case make you feel? Could you personally relate to any of the decision-making filters used by the counselors? Although you may consider some of the sexual and moral dynamics extreme, how are the lessons from their stories instructive for you?

► Case Study 1

John is 32 and divorced. He was married when he turned 20, and that marriage lasted eight years. When asked about his sex life during his marriage, he responds that he and his wife were active sexually during the entire marriage. The divorce was difficult on John. He became a relational recluse for about a year. During that time he was celibate by choice. "In fact," he says, "I didn't even touch anyone."

In the past four years that John has been dating, however, he's found himself in a constant quandary. Because he is good-looking and outgoing, John meets women easily. Though he's never done much introspective work, John is aware of his lingering sense of insecurity about women and tries hard to make a good impression. He wants women to like him. He sees his connections with women as the development of friendships.

Invariably, however, he begins to date his new-found friends and expresses surprise that he becomes sexually involved with them on the second or third date, sometimes the first, usually to the extent of intercourse. When that happens, he begins to withdraw from them, feeling angry at himself for being so undisciplined. Wanting some help in his quandary, he comes to you.

What should he do?

► Case Study 2

Susan has never been married. At age 27, she is proud of her education and accomplishments and the position she has attained as art director at a local advertising agency. Sometimes she stops to think about her singleness and why she has never been involved in any serious relationships since college. But most of the time she keeps busy with work and her social calendar, which includes a church young adult group "when I have the time to go," she adds. Men seem to be attracted to her, but they are also reluctant to ask her out. "Maybe I intimidate them," Susan wonders. "But I'm not really in the mood to pursue anyone, so it's okay with me."

Over the past 18 months, Susan has been involved in three different dating relationships—all of them following the same scenario. All three men have been overanxious. "It's like they wanted to own me," she states. And within four to six weeks, Susan feels an ultimatum: "To bed or bust." She has done both and hates herself for both decisions. For some reason, she also feels responsible for the demise of all the relationships.

What should she do?

► Case Study 3

"We met at work," explains Barbara, a second-year lawyer in a prestigious urban firm. In her business suit she looks more mature than most women at the age of 30. "His name is Robert. He's one of the partners here, and I was his associate for a big case our firm was handling. He didn't put me down or make me feel stupid, and I didn't feel he was trying to get me into bed. I don't know how to interpret it, but our friendship turned into an affair." This was a real surprise to Barbara, who insists she made no conscious choice for a sexual relationship.

Ironically, she says: "I felt no guilt. Besides, his marriage was bad, and I helped him through a tough time." It was her first affair, and she enjoyed it even though she was afraid to admit it. It made her feel safe. She no longer had to worry about the push-and-pull relationship dynamics she experienced with single men who wanted to "smother" her. "Besides," she adds, "there are no good men for someone like me. Every man I meet who is halfway decent is either married, unavailable or gay."

It was after the affair passed its one year anniversary when Barbara began to see things differently. The enjoyment began to wear off. The realization that Robert wasn't going to leave his wife and that she was stuck as the "other woman" was getting old. She tried four or five times to end the relationship, but each time she relented to pressure from Robert and continued to see him. "I want to quit," she declares, "but it seems like I can't. Besides, what are my choices?"

What should Barbara do?

At the same time, Robert is confronted with his duplicity. Finding some receipts from a weekend away with Barbara (supposedly a business trip), Robert's wife, Trish, gives him an ultimatum. "It's her, or me and the kids."

Frightened enough to stop and evaluate his situation, Robert comes to you, his friend. "She's said the same thing before (there was a previous affair). She didn't really mean it then, but now I think she's serious."

What do you tell Robert?

▶ *Case Study 4*

Tom is 26 and has never been married. Always the overachiever in his family, he has compensated for any insecurity by being the best at everything he does. Graduating magna cum laude in both college and graduate school, Tom earned his master's degree in business by age 23. Already moving up the corporate ladder at his company, an international trading firm, Tom earns $50,000 a year and expects his next promotion soon.

His dating life over the past six years has been sporadic at best. "I've never been emotionally close to a woman, and I'm still a virgin," Tom says as he describes his relationships, adding, "at least technically." Six months ago he began a relationship with a woman, a relationship that was obviously different from the others that had preceded it. "I really care for her, and we're at the point where it's commitment time. I know she wants to get married, and so do I, but it's all so scary."

At that point Tom shares his deeper struggle. For the past eight years he has masturbated regularly, a minimum of four times a week, and sometimes as often as two or three times a day. He feels guilty about his secret life and is sure that somehow God is going to punish him. Up to this point he has avoided facing the intense emotional tension and pain caused by his obsession by keeping busy and productive. His hope is that when he consummates a sexual union with his current girlfriend, his problem with masturbation will be solved.

What should he do?

▶ Case Study 5

Anne is 34 and divorced. Only in the past few years has her problem surfaced with such emotional trauma. Anne says she is a lesbian, but is reluctant to go public with her sexual preference. She was aware of her tendency toward the same sex at an early age. And until her early 20s, she had no physical and little emotional contact with men. At age 22, Anne converted to the Christian faith. After her conversion, she shared her story with a church counselor who told her it would be important for her to marry and have children in order to reshape her sexual orientation.

In response to her conversion and the teaching of her church, Anne felt there was a nagging conflict between her faith and her sexual orientation. She did marry at age 24 but was divorced two years later due to unfulfilled desires. "I married him because he was safe," Anne recalls, "but that wasn't a good enough reason for a relationship."

Her relationships since her divorce have been a mixture of both heterosexual and homosexual, although for the last two years she's been celibate. She is currently living with another woman. "At one time," Anne tells the story, "we were emotionally involved with one another. But both of us have made the decision to live a celibate life, yet still live together. Unfortunately, my church has taken exception to my living arrangements. When Sally started coming to church with me, one of the pastors asked if he could talk with us." Told by the church that her lifestyle is immoral, Anne is faced with a choice.

What should she do?

▶ Case Study 6

Steve and Martha have been married for 12 years. Both are 35 years old. Steve is a foreman at a local plant, and Martha has spent the last nine years as a full-time homemaker with three children, ages 9, 5 and 2. For both Steve and Martha, their marriage has provided their only genital sexual relationship. Due to a general sense of unrest, both have decided to come for marital counseling. Their initial sessions are individual and unfold each person's side of the story.

Steve complains that he doesn't get enough sex at home. He says Martha is cold and mechanical when they're in bed. Sometimes during intercourse he finds his mind wandering, and he fantasizes about a woman he knows at work. Although he has expressed anger at Martha for her aloof nature, he has never talked with her about his fantasy life. He believes his fantasies would disappear if his wife cared more about sex.

Martha says she finds sex with Steve okay, but concedes that she has never really enjoyed intercourse and doesn't remember if she's ever experienced an orgasm. Sex, to Martha, is a duty. When asked about her daily routine, Martha remarks that she regularly immerses herself in romance novels. "They're a wonderful escape from my daily routine," she explains. "Besides, the feelings I have when I read them make me feel romantic and special. I've never felt that way with Steve." On their next session, they come as a couple.

What should they do?

▶ Case Study 7

Rick is 27 and married. He and his wife, Linda, have been married for five years, but as of yet, have no children. Rick has an influential management position in a large Christian parachurch agency. He is happy with his job and hopes he can continue in his field for another 10 to 20 years. Linda is also a career professional, working as a clothing line representative for a department store chain. Rick describes their marriage as good. "We're compatible, and we still enjoy each other's company," he comments.

Rick's dilemma? For the past four years, he has been hooked on pornography. "It started with magazines," he recalls, "but it wasn't long before I was going to peep shows and adult bookstores, at least once or twice a month. Linda doesn't know, and I can't tell anyone at church. Sometimes the urge gets worse, and sometimes it doesn't seem to bother me at all. I try not to think about what I'm doing; it all seems so reprehensible. But it's like a fix, even though I feel awful afterward. I want to quit, but I just don't know how."

What should he do?

An Afterword

The temptation lingers. I've just reread the book and am hit again with the questions: "But what have we resolved here?" "Have we answered all the questions?" "Have I said enough?" "Have I said too much?" It's a persistent reminder that I too am a product of the Michelob generation. "Who says you can't have it all?"

We want the issue resolved. Okay, I confess, *I* want the issue resolved. I want answers. I want comfort. Or, at least, I want to feel that we have partially accomplished the cultural call to feel good about our sexuality. Somehow it's not enough just to raise the issue, to create an environment for dialogue, to learn to ask the right questions and to join in the struggle.

So, I guess if all your questions were answered, I didn't do my job. The illusion of closure only leads us to further isolation and assumed self-sufficiency. It is our ambiguity that keeps us in community. Because we don't have all the answers, we need to continue to talk to each other and to God—to ask, doubt, learn and grow.

In the flurry and emotional momentum of this already overburdened subject, is there permission to struggle with the issue, an invitation to experience forgiveness and a light of hope at the end of the tunnel? Is there permission to believe that mixed emotions are okay? I believe the answers are yes. Someday I hope that my ambivalence and pain in the area of sexuality will subside. But even if they don't, I want to learn that it's okay to live with these feelings and that my emotions are user-friendly.

I will confess that many of my arguments were carried to an extreme, especially on the issue of grace. (I suspect that God's grace is far more outrageous.) But I'm also willing to live with that. For if I'm going to err, I would much rather err on the side of grace.

As I wrote, I was struck with three recurring themes. The first was my continuing temptation to temper the issue of grace with some carefully worded disclaimers, my own version of a "Yes . . . but . . ." theology. Grace still makes me uncomfortable; I'm far more comfortable as a legalist or a narcissist depending upon my mood.

The second theme was the persistent throbbing of grace. Ironically, the issue of morality is not dependent upon our final word or conclusion about ourselves, or our conclusion about grace for that matter. Beyond our discussions and our feeble attempts at theology and self-justification is God's word about us—his relentless, passionate affirmation of our value and his unfaltering commitment to our well-being.

And the third theme was the ever-present, overriding seriousness and paranoia that accompanies almost any discussion on the subject of sexuality. It's apparent we take ourselves far too seriously. It wouldn't hurt for us to stop and laugh at ourselves—at our expertise, at our fear and at our need to make life nice and neat.

I remember my pastor, Ben Patterson, saying: "Humor can strip away pretense and illusion . . . Like anything human, it is a gift from God filled with wonder and mystery. Also, like anything human, it is just that: human, mortal, ephemeral. In the resurrection there will be no marriage, said Jesus. We were not made for our appetites, but for the Lord, said Paul. Christians, who tend to ascribe to sex nearly unlimited power of destruction, need to have a good belly laugh over playful eros. Others, who would make a good lay the end of all human existence, need also to see the disparity between what the claims of sex are and what it actually delivers. And laugh until they cry."

There is much more to be written and learned about the subject of sexuality and the choices we make. But maybe a little humor will help us with our perspective. Since our fear distorts the subject of morality, our humor may help to expose our fear as overprotective and controlling. In our need to be right, relevant, in control or spiritual, we can easily miss the point that joy comes with the celebration of life and the sanctity of relationships.

Notes

Preface

[1] Arnold Lobel, *Frog and Toad Together* (New York: Harper & Row, 1971), 30-41.

[2] Pat Conroy, *The Prince of Tides* (New York: Bantam, 1987), 294.

[3] Frederick Buechner, *Wishful Thinking* (San Francisco: Harper & Row, 1973), 87.

[4] Lewis Smedes, *Sex for Christians* (San Francisco: Eerdmans, 1976), 9-10.

Section One: Introduction

[1] Susan Littwin, *The Postponed Generation* (New York: Morrow, 1987), 15-16.

[2] Gail Sheehy, *Passages* (New York: E.P. Dutton & Co., 1976), 28.

[3] Littwin, *The Postponed Generation*, 22.

Chapter 1

[1] Robert N. Bellah et. al., *Habits of the Heart* (Berkeley: University of California, 1985), 65.

[2] Susan Littwin, *The Postponed Generation* (New York: Morrow, 1987), 215.

[3] Betty Cuniberti, "Yuppie Angst: Coping With Stress of Success," *Los Angeles Times* (November 21, 1986), 1.

[4] Bellah et. al., *Habits of the Heart*, 139.

[5] Littwin, *The Postponed Generation*, 230.

[6] Harold Kushner, *When All You've Ever Wanted Isn't Enough* (New York: Summit, 1986), 61.

[7] Beth Ann Krier, "The Essence of Cocooning," *Los Angeles Times* (August 7, 1987), 1.

[8] George Leonard, *The End of Sex* (Los Angeles: Tarcher, 1983), 10.

9 Quoted in Lorna and Philip Sarrel, "The Death of Lust in an Age of Easy Virtue," GQ (August 1984), 122.

Chapter 2

1 Eugene Kennedy, *The Trouble With Being Human*, (New York: Doubleday, 1986), 75.

2 Quoted in Lee Eisenberg, "The Master Plan," Esquire (May 1987), 15.

3 Kennedy, *The Trouble With Being Human*, 81.

4 Andrew Greeley, *Sexual Intimacy* (New York: Harper & Row, 1975), 45.

5 George Leonard, *The End of Sex* (Los Angeles: Tarcher, 1983), 203.

6 Greeley, *Sexual Intimacy*, 37, 41.

Chapter 3

1 Henri Nouwen, *Making All Things New* (New York: Harper & Row, 1981), 36.

2 C.S. Lewis, *Mere Christianity* (New York: Macmillan, 1943), 161.

3 Gabrielle Brown, *The New Celibacy* (New York: Ballantine, 1980), 161.

4 Andrew Greeley, *Sexual Intimacy* (New York: Harper & Row, 1975), 81.

5 William Lenters, *The Freedom We Crave* (Grand Rapids, MI: Eerdmans, 1985), viii.

6 Anne Wilson Schaef, *Co-Dependence*, (San Francisco: Harper & Row, 1986), 21.

7 Lenters, *The Freedom We Crave*, 4.

8 Lenters, *The Freedom We Crave*, 19.

9 Lenters, *The Freedom We Crave*, 9.

10 Eugene Kennedy, *Sexual Counseling* (New York: Continuum, 1980), 112.

11 Howard M. Halpern, *How to Break Your Addiction to a Person* (New York: Bantam, 1987), 2.

12 Merle Shain, *When Lovers Are Friends* (New York: Bantam, 1980), 84.

13 James Sennett, "The Myth of Consistency," The Wittenburg Door (December 1984-January 1985), 3.

14 Merle Shain, *Some Men Are More Perfect Than Others* (New York: Bantam, 1980), 39.

Chapter 4

[1] Lewis Smedes, *Sex for Christians* (Grand Rapids, MI: Eerdmans, 1976), 24.

[2] Eugene Kennedy, *The Trouble With Being Human* (New York: Doubleday, 1986), 14.

[3] Sam Keen, *The Passionate Life* (San Francisco: Harper & Row, 1983), 49.

[4] Keen, *The Passionate Life*, 140.

[5] Keen, *The Passionate Life*, 190-191.

[6] Keith Clark, *Being Sexual . . . and Celibate* (Notre Dame: Ave Maria, 1986), 56.

[7] Anthony DeMello, *The Song of the Bird* (New York: Doubleday, 1984), 65-66.

[8] James Carroll, *Prince of Peace* (New York: Signet, 1985), 482.

[9] Morton Kelsey and Barbara Kelsey, *Sacrament of Sexuality* (Warwick, NY: Amity House, 1986), 80.

Chapter 5

[1] Morton Kelsey and Barbara Kelsey, *Sacrament of Sexuality* (Warwick, NY: Amity House, 1986), 5.

[2] Kelsey and Kelsey, *Sacrament of Sexuality*, 103.

[3] Andrew Greeley, *Sexual Intimacy* (New York: Harper & Row, 1975), 186.

[4] Mel White, *The Other Side of Love* (Old Tappan, NJ: Revell, 1978), 25.

[5] Kelsey and Kelsey, *Sacrament of Sexuality*, 28.

[6] Kelsey and Kelsey, *Sacrament of Sexuality*, 29.

[7] Donald Nicholl, *Holiness* (New York: Harper & Row, 1981), 46.

[8] Harold Kushner, *When All You've Ever Wanted Isn't Enough* (New York: Summit, 1986), 81-82.

[9] Lewis Smedes, *Sex for Christians* (San Francisco: Eerdmans, 1976), 30.

[10] Greeley, *Sexual Intimacy*, 64-65.

[11] Kushner, *When All You've Ever Wanted Isn't Enough*, 82-83.

Chapter 6

[1] Andrew Greeley, *Sexual Intimacy* (New York: Harper

& Row, 1975), 37.

[2] Mel White, *The Other Side of Love* (Old Tappan, NJ: Revell, 1978), 33.

[3] Lewis Smedes, *Mere Morality* (Grand Rapids, MI: Eerdmans, 1987), 10.

[4] Frederick Buechner, *Wishful Thinking* (San Francisco: Harper & Row, 1973), 63-64.

[5] Smedes, *Mere Morality*, 8.

[6] George Leonard, *The End of Sex* (Los Angeles: Tarcher, 1983), 168.

[7] Keith Clark, *Being Sexual . . . and Celibate* (Notre Dame: Ave Maria, 1986), 79.

[8] Greeley, *Sexual Intimacy*, 163.

[9] Smedes, *Mere Morality*, 13.

Section Three: Introduction

[1] Morris West, *Cassidy* (New York: Doubleday, 1986), 89.

Chapter 7

[1] Keith Clark, *Being Sexual . . . and Celibate* (Notre Dame: Ave Maria, 1986), 77.

[2] Clark, *Being Sexual . . . and Celibate*, 87.

[3] Eugene Kennedy, *The Trouble With Being Human* (New York: Doubleday, 1986), 139.

[4] C.S. Lewis, *The Weight of Glory* (Grand Rapids, MI: Eerdmans, 1979), 15.

[5] Andrew Greeley, *Sexual Intimacy* (New York: Harper & Row, 1975), 56.

[6] Robert N. Bellah et. al., *Habits of the Heart* (Berkeley: University of California, 1985), 93.

[7] Kennedy, *The Trouble With Being Human*, 84.

[8] C.S. Lewis, *Mere Christianity* (New York: Macmillan, 1943), 90-93.

[9] Judith Viorst, *Necessary Losses* (New York: Simon and Schuster, 1986), 16.

[10] Quoted in Keith Clark, *An Experience of Celibacy* (Notre Dame: Ave Maria, 1982), 102.

[11] Peter Kreitler, *Affair Prevention* (New York: Macmillan, 1981), 124.

[12] Lewis Smedes, *Choices* (San Francisco: Harper & Row, 1986), 70.

[13] Clark, *An Experience of Celibacy*, 103.

[14] Greeley, *Sexual Intimacy*, 188.

Chapter 8

[1] Lewis Smedes, *Choices* (San Francisco: Harper & Row, 1986), 64.

[2] Smedes *Choices*, 65.

[3] Harold Kushner, *When All You've Ever Wanted Isn't Enough* (New York: Summit, 1986), 123.

[4] Nancy Weber, "Unfaithfully Yours," GQ (August 1986), 79-80.

[5] Walter Shapiro, "What's Wrong," Time (May 25, 1987), 16.

[6] Robert F. Capon, *Between Noon and Three* (San Francisco: Harper & Row, 1982), 148.

[7] Robert F. Capon, "Pietro and Madeleine," Wittenburg Door (April 1986-May 1986), 9.

[8] Kushner, *When All You've Ever Wanted Isn't Enough*, 132.

Chapter 9

[1] Laurel Richardson, *The New Other Woman* (New York: Free Press, 1987), 84.

[2] Alice Miller, *The Drama of the Gifted Child* (New York: Basic, 1983), ix.

[3] Harold Kushner, *When All You've Ever Wanted Isn't Enough* (New York: Summit, 1986), 62.

[4] Robert N. Bellah et. al., *Habits of the Heart* (Berkeley: University of California, 1985), 129.

[5] Peter Kreitler, *Affair Prevention* (New York: Macmillan, 1981), 65.

[6] Kushner, *When All You've Ever Wanted Isn't Enough*, 62.

[7] Kushner, *When All You've Ever Wanted Isn't Enough*, 63.

[8] Tim Stafford, "Great Sex: Reclaiming a Christian Sexual Ethic," Christianity Today (October 2, 1987), 36.

[9] Quoted in John White, "Wait Awhile," His (May

1981), 7.
[10] Quoted in White, "Wait Awhile," 7.

Chapter 10

[1] Morris West, *Cassidy* (New York: Doubleday, 1986), 153.

[2] Lewis Smedes, *Choices* (San Francisco: Harper & Row, 1986), 79.

[3] Viktor E. Frankl, *The Unheard Cry for Meaning* (New York: Simon and Schuster, 1978), 56.

[4] Robert F. Capon, *Between Noon and Three* (San Francisco: Harper & Row, 1982), 174.

[5] Harold Kushner, *When All You've Ever Wanted Isn't Enough* (New York: Summit, 1986), 135-136.

[6] Capon, *Between Noon and Three*, 112.

[7] Capon, *Between Noon and Three*, 112.

[8] Capon, *Between Noon and Three*, 109.

[9] "The Wittenburg Door Interview: Brennan Manning," The Wittenburg Door (October 1986-November 1986), 15.

[10] Keith Miller and Andrea Wells Miller, *The Single Experience* (Waco, TX: Word, 1981), 228.

[11] Lewis Smedes, *Sex for Christians* (San Francisco: Eerdmans, 1976), 88.

[12] Keith Clark, *Being Sexual . . . and Celibate* (Notre Dame: Ave Maria, 1986), 104.

[13] These questions are based on Smedes, *Choices*, 95-114.

[14] Smedes, *Choices*, 104-105.

[15] "The Wittenburg Door Interview: Brennan Manning," 17.

Chapter 11

[1] Lewis Smedes, *Choices* (San Francisco: Harper & Row, 1986), 121.

[2] Robert F. Capon, *Between Noon and Three* (San Francisco: Harper & Row, 1982), 172.

[3] Capon, *Between Noon and Three*, 157.

[4] Capon, *Between Noon and Three*, 119.

[5] Robert F. Capon, "Pietro and Madeleine," Wittenburg Door (April 1985-May 1985), 22.

6 Robert F. Capon, *The Parables of the Kingdom* (Grand Rapids, MI: Zondervan, 1985), 84.

7 Philip Yancey, "The Shape of God's Body," Leadership (Summer 1987), 94.

8 Robert F. Capon, "Pietro and Madeleine," Wittenburg Door (April 1986-May 1986), 9.

9 Capon, *Between Noon and Three*, 8.

10 Smedes, *Choices*, 121.

Section Four: Introduction

1 Merle Shain, *When Lovers Are Friends* (New York: Bantam, 1980), 83.

2 Shain, *When Lovers Are Friends*, 74-75.

Chapter 12

1 Andrew Greeley, *Sexual Intimacy* (New York: Harper & Row, 1975), 60.

2 Keith Miller and Andrea Wells Miller, *The Single Experience* (Waco, TX: Word, 1981), 228.

3 Terry Hershey, *Young Adult Ministry* (Loveland, CO: Group, 1986), 42.

4 Eugene Kennedy, *The Trouble With Being Human* (New York: Doubleday, 1986), 113.

5 Kennedy, *The Trouble With Being Human*, 117.

6 Greeley, *Sexual Intimacy*, 60.

7 Quoted in Benedict J. Groeschel, *The Courage to Be Chaste* (Mahwah, NJ: Paulist, 1985), 93.

8 C.S. Lewis, *Mere Christianity* (New York: Macmillan, 1943), 93-94.

9 Susan Littwin, *The Postponed Generation* (New York: Morrow, 1987), 247.

10 Robert F. Capon, *Between Noon and Three* (San Francisco: Harper & Row, 1982), 176.

Bibliography

Bellah, Robert N. et al. *Habits of the Heart*. Berkeley: University of California, 1985.

Bonhoeffer, Dietrich. *Ethics*. New York: Macmillan, 1965.

Brown, Gabrielle. *The New Celibacy*. New York: McGraw-Hill, 1980.

Buechner, Frederick. *Wishful Thinking*. San Francisco: Harper & Row, 1973.

Capon, Robert F. *Between Noon and Three*. San Francisco: Harper & Row, 1982.

Capon, Robert F. *The Parables of the Kingdom*. Grand Rapids, MI: Zondervan, 1985.

Carnes, Patrick. *Out of the Shadows: Understanding Sexual Addiction*. Minneapolis: CompCare, 1985.

Clark, Keith. *An Experience of Celibacy*. Notre Dame: Ave Maria, 1982.

Clark, Keith. *Being Sexual . . . and Celibate*. Notre Dame: Ave Maria, 1986.

DeMello, Anthony. *The Song of the Bird*. New York: Doubleday, 1984.

Foster, Richard. *Money, Sex & Power*. San Francisco: Harper & Row, 1985.

Frankl, Viktor E. *The Unheard Cry for Meaning*. New York: Simon and Schuster, 1978.

Gilder, George. *Men and Marriage*, rev. ed. Gretna, LA: Pelican, 1986.

Goergen, Don. *The Sexual Celibate*. New York: Harper & Row, 1975.

Greeley, Andrew. *Sexual Intimacy*. New York: Harper & Row, 1975.

Groeschel, Benedict J. *The Courage to Be Chaste*. Mahwah, NJ: Paulist, 1985.

Hershey, Terry. *Beginning Again*. Nashville: Thomas Nelson, 1986.

Hershey, Terry. *Intimacy: The Longing of Every Human Heart*. Eugene, OR: Harvest House, 1984.

Hershey, Terry. *Young Adult Ministry*. Loveland, CO: Group, 1986.

Johnson, Robert A. *We*. San Francisco: Harper & Row, 1983.

Keen, Sam. *The Passionate Life*. San Francisco: Harper & Row, 1983.

Kelsey, Morton and Kelsey, Barbara. *Sacrament of Sexuality*. Warwick, NY: Amity House, 1986.

Kennedy, Eugene. *Sexual Counseling*. New York: Continuum, 1980.

Kennedy, Eugene. *The Trouble With Being Human*. New York: Doubleday, 1986.

Kreitler, Peter. *Affair Prevention*. New York: Macmillan, 1981.

Kushner, Harold. *When All You've Ever Wanted Isn't Enough*. New York: Summit, 1986.

Lenters, William. *The Freedom We Crave*. Grand Rapids, MI: Eerdmans, 1985.

Leonard, George. *The End of Sex*. Los Angeles: Tarcher, 1983.

Lewis, C.S. *Christian Reflections*. Grand Rapids, MI: Eerdmans, 1974.

Lewis, C.S. *God in the Dock*. Grand Rapids, MI: Eerdmans, 1970.

Lewis, C.S. *Mere Christianity*. New York: Macmillan, 1943.

Littwin, Susan. *The Postponed Generation*. New York: Morrow, 1987.

McGinnis, Alan L. *The Friendship Factor*. Minneapolis: Augsburg, 1979.

Miller, Keith and Miller, Andrea Wells. *The Single Experience*. Waco, TX: Word, 1981.

Muto, Susan Annette. *Celebrating the Single Life*. New York: Doubleday, 1982.

Peck, M. Scott. *The Road Less Traveled*. New York: Simon and Schuster, 1980.

Richardson, Laurel. *The New Other Woman*. New York: Free Press, 1987.

Schaef, Anne Wilson *Co-Dependence*. San Francisco: Harper & Row, 1986.

Shain, Merle. *Some Men Are More Perfect Than Others*. New York: Bantam, 1980.

Shain, Merle. *When Lovers Are Friends*. New York: Bantam, 1980.

Smedes, Lewis. *Choices*. San Francisco: Harper & Row, 1986.

Smedes, Lewis. *Mere Morality*. Grand Rapids, MI: Eerdmans, 1987.

Smedes, Lewis. *Sex for Christians*. Grand Rapids, MI: Eerdmans, 1976.

Viorst, Judith. *Necessary Losses*. New York: Simon and Schuster, 1986.

White, John. *Eros Defiled*. Downers Grove, IL: InterVarsity, 1977.

White, Mel. *The Other Side of Love*. Old Tappan, NJ: Revell, 1978.

Terry Hershey is executive director of Christian Focus Inc., a ministry committed to building and nurturing healthy relationships. He is available for seminars, conferences and consultations for your church or organization. In addition, he has produced other books and tape series that may benefit you or your church.

His seminar subjects include:

► Intimacy: Building Healthy Relationships
► Young Adult Ministry
► Beginning Again: Life After a Relationship Ends
► Clear-Headed Choices in a Sexually Confused World
► Slowing Down in a Hurry-Up World
► Developing Leadership and Giving the Church Away

For more information on other Christian Focus ministries or other books and tapes by Terry Hershey, please call or write:

Christian Focus Inc.
Box 17134
Irvine, CA 92713
(714) 756-1911